Parallel Imports of Pharmaceuticals

Evidence from Scandinavia and Policy
Proposals for Switzerland

by Cédric Julien Poget

Birkhäuser
Basel · Boston · Berlin

Cédric Julien Poget
WWZ
Basel University
Petersgraben 51
CH-4003 Basel

Library of Congress Control Number: 2007935341

Bibliographic information published by Die Deutsche Bibliothek
Die Deutsche Bibliothek lists this publication in the Deutsche Nationalbibliografie;
detailed bibliographic data is available in the Internet at <http://dnb.ddb.de>.

ISBN 978-3-7643-8588-0   Birkhäuser Verlag AG, Basel – Boston – Berlin

© 2008 Birkhäuser Verlag AG, P.O. Box 133, CH-4010 Basel, Switzerland
Part of Springer Science+Business Media
Printed on acid-free paper produced from chlorine-free pulp. TCF ∞
Cover design: Alexander Faust, Basel, Switzerland
Printed in Germany

ISBN 978-3-7643-8588-0   e-ISBN 978-3-7643-8589-7

9 8 7 6 5 4 3 2 1   www.birkhauser.ch

Contents

Tables

Figures

Acknowledgements

It is both a great pleasure and an honour for me to thank all the people who have supported me throughout my PhD project and so contributed to my bringing it to a successful end.

I express my deep gratitude to Prof. Dr. Jürg Sommer, who offered me a position in his department and supported me with continuous counsel and advice. He taught me how to focus my research and gave me outstanding guidance during the whole project. I would also like to thank Prof. Dr. Rolf Weder for accepting to be the second reviewer.

I am very grateful to Interpharma and Thomas Cueni for supporting me with a grant and expert counsel and making possible several international journeys which were necessary to meet the experts involved with parallel trade. This allowed me to deepen my understanding of the relevant pharmaceutical markets, parallel trade and the healthcare sector at large.

The data which were needed to accomplish my empirical analyses came from Dansk Lægemiddel Information, Läkemedelsstatistik (Sweden) and Farmastat (Norway). My special gratitude is due to Jørgen Clausen at Lif Denmark, Olle Hagberg at Lif and Erik Stene at LMI for helping me to gain access to market data in Scandinavia. I also would like to extend my thanks to all my interview partners and market insight providers who helped me to acquire the knowledge that specialized literature would not offer, namely

Association of the British Pharmaceutical Industry (ABPI): Phil O'Neill
Bayer AG: Dirk Ehle and Engelbert Gith
Eurim-Pharm: Andreas Mohringer
EFPIA: François Bouvy
Farmindustria (España): Iciar Sanz de Madrid
Farmindustria (Italia): Antonella Moroni
F. Hoffmann-La Roche AG: Peter Heer, René Imhof and Hans-Ruedi Wiedmer
Interpharma: SibylleAugsburger, Thomas Cueni, Mercedes Montoro, Dominique Reinhard, Heiner Sandmeier, Vincenza Trivigno and Raphaël Tschanz
Lægemiddelindustriforeningen (Lif DK): Jørgen Clausen
Läkemedelsindustriföreningen, (LIF): Olle Hageberg, Margita Jacobsson and Mats Ollson
Legemiddelindsutrieforenigen (LMI): Erik A. Stene and Per Olav Kormeset
LEEM: Valérie Béquart, François-Regis Moulines and Béatrice Kressman
Leo-Pharma: Jesper Noerregard
Novartis AG: Martin Batzer, Ernst Buser and Stephan Mumenthaler
Orifarm (Danmark) A/S: Thomas Brandhof, Ulrik Markussen and Hans Bøgh-Sørensen
Orifarm (Sverige) AB: Fredrik Persson
Pharos: Theo Berendsen
SFEE: Yannis Chryssospathis
Roche Deutschland Holding GmbH: Alexander Keusgen, Karl Schlingensief
Roche Diagnostics (Deutschland) GmbH: Wulf-Fischer Knuppertz
UCB Pharma: Simon Loomann, Christian Matton and Egdar Theusinger
Verband Forschender Arzneimittelhersteller (VFA): Walter Wittig

Finally I would like to thank my colleagues here at the faculty of economics for many enriching conversations and Pauline Baumgartner, Jacqui Hutteman and Josh Merrill for their counsel on English language, style and grammar. I thank my parents, friends and all other persons who encouraged and helped me in the course of my work.

My apologies if I have inadvertently omitted anyone to whom acknowledgement is due.

Basle, May 21st, 2007
Cédric Poget

1

Introduction to parallel trade

Parallel traded goods are genuine products brought into a market without prior authorisation of the intellectual property right or trademark holder. Parallel trade occurs if international price differences for identical products are high and a policy of regional or international exhaustion of the respective property right has been implemented in the high price country. In a world without trade barriers, prices converge to a global equilibrium, provided transaction costs are nil and competition among arbitrage seekers is perfect. The price convergence benefits consumers in the high demand country who are able to increase their private consumption as prices go down. Consumers in the low demand country, on the other hand, lose as rising prices force them to lower their consumption. Global consumer surplus is generally higher under uniform pricing than under price discrimination. Generally – because consumers in the low demand country may not be able to afford the world market price. Under such circumstances, consumers in the high demand country end up paying the price which would have been charged under market segmentation, while consumers in the low demand country are unable to buy the product. International exhaustion of property rights may, therefore, reduce global welfare if income disparities are high. Representatives of the drug industry argue that parallel trade reduces global welfare by impairing their ability to develop new products. Allowing parallel imports of pharmaceuticals would therefore be a trade-off between immediate and future customer value. If savings from parallel trade are high and research efficiency of the industry is low, governments should opt for a policy of international or regional exhaustion. If savings are low and research efficiency high, however, national exhaustion of patent rights would be the appropriate policy.

In the European Union, regional exhaustion of intellectual property rights was cemented in 1974 by the European Court of Justice in a prominent lawsuit between Centrafarm BV and Sterling Drug Inc[1]. Ever since parallel trade volumes have been growing faster than the overall market and parallel traders are now holding market shares between six and thirteen percent in the six major destination markets.

This report analyses how parallel imports of pharmaceuticals are affecting end consumer prices and drug expenditures in three Scandinavian countries, Sweden, Denmark and Norway. It finds that patient/pharmacist incentives to switch to a lower priced product are an important factor in determining savings from parallel trade. Sweden, for instance, has achieved sizeable savings both from generic and from parallel traded competition by requiring pharmacists to always dispense the cheapest product and by limiting the reimbursement price to that same level. In Norway, however, savings are low, because patients lack incentives to switch to a lower priced product. Moreover, Norwegian wholesalers are

---

1   ECJ Judgement on the case 15/74, available on: www.curia.eu.int (Accessed on 15.01.2005)

able to retain a substantial share of the price difference between the locally sourced and the parallel traded drug.

In the last chapter we discuss how Switzerland could benefit from allowing parallel trade of pharmaceuticals. By using market shares and prices of parallel traded products observed in Europe as a reference, we develop a set of estimates for the impact that allowing parallel trade would have on Swiss consumers. Based on our findings, we develop policy proposals for Switzerland and Europe.

2

Parallel trade of pharmaceuticals in Norway

2.1   Summary

Before Norway joined the European Economic Area in 1994, parallel imports of pharmaceuticals were not permitted. In the first year of its membership Norway allowed parallel imports of non-patented drugs. Parallel imports of patented pharmaceuticals became legal in 1995[2]. The high price level and financial incentives to the pharmacist allowed parallel importers to penetrate the market quickly and market shares hit 7.7% in 2000. Because of substantial price cuts on branded drugs which were imposed by the Norwegian government, market shares of parallel traded products eased back to 5.1% in the year 2002[3]. In 2005 market shares of parallel traded pharmaceuticals were back at 6.9%[4]. Research on 25 top selling pharmaceuticals reveals that the average parallel traded pharmaceutical was priced 3% below the locally sourced drug between October 2003 and September 2004. Parallel imported drugs have cut overall drug expenditures by 0.2%. Norway is the Scandinavian country where price advantages and market shares of parallel traded drugs are the lowest.

This chapter shows why patient savings from parallel traded drugs are relatively low in Norway, and closes with policy recommendations for driving consumer savings up and distribution mark-ups down.

2.2   The Norwegian healthcare system

2.2.1   Organization

Healthcare in Norway is funded through taxation, by the government. The central government defines, implements and supervises healthcare laws and regulations. Municipalities receive block grants from the central government for providing healthcare, education and infrastructure for the population. It is in the local governments responsibility to prioritize among different services. Savings achieved in healthcare can be used to finance other projects and vice versa[5].

---

2   Bouvy F (2003) Overview of pricing and reimbursement measures taken since January 1993, Working Document, EFPIA, Brussels

3   LMI (2007), Facts and Figures 2007: Medicines and Healthcare, P. 37, Oslo, Norway

4   LMI (2007), Facts and Figures 2007: Medicines and Healthcare, P. 37, Oslo, Norway

5   Roth Johnsen J (2006), Health Systems in Transition: Norway, Volume 8 No. 1, 2006, Page 63

In Norway general practitioners have a gate keeping function. Moreover, they are responsible for providing basic healthcare services for the population. Only authorised and licensed physicians can have their services reimbursed by the national insurance system. The general practitioners compensation model has three elements[6]:
1. A per capita payment for every registered patient
2. Fee for service reimbursement for each consultation, with different rates for different types of consultations
3. Co-payments from patients for each consultation, with different rates for different consultations

Fixed per capita reimbursement represents 30% of a physician's income. Activity based compensations and co-payments amount to 70%[7] of his revenue. Physicians may, therefore, provide unnecessary or inappropriate services to a patient. The threat of having their license removed, however, provides incentives to act inline with the authorities' directives. Limiting the number of general practitioners is a further tool used by municipalities to control and anticipate expenditure on out-patient care.

In 2002, ownership of Norwegian hospitals was transferred to the central government. Each hospital is organized as a private entity and has two sources of finance; lump sum payments and diagnostics related payments for each patient treated. Norwegian hospitals have strong incentives to cure each patient in a cost effective manner. The ownership of all hospitals allows the government to directly influence the capacity of the in-patient sector and its investments in new equipment and technology.

We conclude that the government controls in- and out-patient expenditures through the limitation of the number and the selection of healthcare professionals in primary care, the gate-keeping function of general practitioners and the ownership and control of the hospital market.

Drug manufacturers and parallel traders are privately run, *profit maximizing* businesses. The government cannot dictate to parallel traders which products are to be imported at what price advantage compared to the locally sourced product. Instead, the government has to influence the behaviour of those stakeholders who are prescribing, distributing and buying parallel traded pharmaceuticals. Inducing parallel traders to behave in a desired way is therefore more difficult than inducing government controlled hospitals to do the same thing. In the next subchapters we will look at how successful the government is in influencing stakeholders' behaviour.

2.2.2 Reimbursement of pharmaceuticals

Pharmaceuticals in Norway are divided into three categories: over the counter, white and blue prescription drugs. Over the counter drugs and white prescription medicines are not eligible for reimbursement by the National Insurance System. White prescription drugs are generally used on less serious and temporary conditions. The blue prescription list includes drugs that are considered to be important by the authorities. The majority of all blue listed

---

6   Roth Johnsen J (2006), Health Systems in Transition: Norway, Volume 8 No. 1, 2006, Page 63
7   Roth Johnsen J (2006), Health Systems in Transition: Norway, Volume 8 No. 1, 2006, Page 63

pharmaceuticals are used on chronic diseases, cancer and the palliative medicine. New pharmaceuticals are classified as important whenever providing a clear progress in therapy. Co-payment on blue listed pharmaceuticals is 36% of the pharmacy distribution price, with a per prescription cap of NOK 500.– (EUR 61)[8]. Once a co-payment ceiling of NOK 1 615 (EUR 200) is reached, a card is issued which entitles the patient to receive free treatment and benefits for the remainder of the year.

In the year 2003, patients financed one third of total expenditures for pharmaceuticals out of their own pocket. This is one of the highest shares in Europe. The reason being, that the public health insurance in Norway does not reimburse prescription drugs used on conditions that are not considered to be serious. Reimbursement conditions on blue prescription drugs, however, are favourable, with 91% of total costs being reimbursed by the National Insurance System[9].

This aspect is very important when referring to parallel trade of pharmaceuticals. Later in this chapter, we will see that two thirds of total revenue with parallel traded drugs is generated with the 26 top selling brands in Norway. The majority of these pharmaceuticals is used on chronic conditions such as hypertension, high cholesterol, cancer, asthma and schizophrenia. We recall that important pharmaceuticals used on chronic conditions are the ones that are eligible for reimbursement. Low self contributions on these products reduce a patient's incentive to act cost effectively. This removes some pressure from parallel traders to compete with prices.

2.2.3 The price setting process for pharmaceuticals

The Norwegian Medicines Agency (Statens legemiddelverk/NMA) is the national regulatory authority for new and existing medicines. It regulates prices and trade conditions of pharmaceuticals. Other responsibilities include the supervision of production, trials and marketing of pharmaceuticals and the evaluation and authorisation of new medicines.

Pharmacy purchasing (AIP) and distribution prices (AUP) of pharmaceuticals are set upon registration and adjusted on a regular basis. Ex-factory prices, however, are free. The maximal price of a drug is set at the average of the three lowest prices observed in a selection of countries. Normally, the maximal price is set by reference to the following countries: Austria, Belgium, Finland, Germany, Great Britain, Ireland and the Netherlands[10]. Additionally, the NMA may refer to the pharmacy price observed in Greece, Italy, Portugal, Spain and *Switzerland.*

Wholesalers may charge for product anything which is either at or below the official pharmacy purchasing price (AIP). Pharmacist may price their products up to the official pharmacy distribution price (AUP). Pharmacists, who have obtained a price which is lower than AIP, are requested to reimburse half of the difference between AIP and the effective procurement price to the public health insurance. They can keep the other half for themselves. Pharmacists have therefore strong incentives to buy from the wholesaler who charges the lowest possible price for a product.

8   Roth Johnsen J (2006), Health Systems in Transition: Norway, Volume 8 No. 1, 2006, Page 63

9   EFPIA (2006), The Pharmaceutical Industry in Figures, Page 37, Brussels

10 Roth Johnsen J (2006), Health Systems in Transition: Norway, Volume 8 No. 1, 2006, Page 63

Wholesalers have incentives to buy from the cheapest supplier too because they are entitled to keep the full difference between the price that their supplier charges for a product and the official pharmacy purchasing price. Both wholesalers and pharmacists are therefore expected to buy and distribute parallel traded pharmaceuticals. The Norwegian wholesalers' and pharmacists' compensation system is suitable to induce price competition among parallel traders.

2.2.4   The distribution chain of pharmaceuticals in Norway

a)   Wholesalers

Until 1994, Norsk Medisianldepot (NMD), a government owned wholesaler, held the monopoly for supplying pharmacies and hospitals with pharmaceuticals. When joining the EEA in 1994, Norway was forced to abandon its ownership of NMD. In order to prevent a privatized NMD from abusing its monopoly towards pharmacies and hospitals, two further wholesalers were admitted to the market. NMD was purchased by Celesio, an international wholesaling and retailing conglomerate. In the year 2006, NMD/Celesio controlled 45.6% of the Norwegian drug market followed by Tamro/Phoenix (34.3%) and Holtung (20.1%)[11]. Phoenix, a German company has wholesaling activities in ten and retailing businesses in seven European countries. Holtung is a subsidiary of Alliance Unichem, one of Britain's leading pharmaceutical wholesaling and retailing conglomerates. These wholesalers can, therefore, use the whole market power of their holding companies to negotiate price cuts in Norway.

b)   Pharmacists

Until 2001, the Norwegian Board of Health was responsible for locating pharmacies, so as to adequately cover the whole population[12]. Only pharmacists could own and run a pharmacy. As a consequence, pharmacy chains were virtually nonexistent. A centralized purchasing system, which had been set up in 1996, allowed pharmacists to buy in bulk from the cheapest supplier.

In the year 2001, a law was passed allowing greater freedom to the establishment of pharmacies. It loosened the ownership restrictions for pharmacies, allowing anyone, except physicians and pharmaceutical companies, to own a pharmacy. Wholesalers responded by taking over the majority of the retail market. Their margins had come under heavy pressure when, in 1996, more than 90% of all pharmacies had been linked up to a centralized purchasing system. To understand the rationale behind the acquisition strategy, let us compare how independent and affiliated pharmacies make their purchasing decisions. Independent pharmacies will always buy from the cheapest supplier, thus forcing wholesalers to gradually reduce their distribution margins. Affiliated pharmacies, however, will now buy a more expensive product from the wholesaler they are affiliated to, if doing so maximises profits of the wholesaling corporation. We observe that this sum is generally maximized if wholesalers supply their own pharmacies. The following example helps to understand why:

---

11   LMI (2007), Facts and Figures 2007: Medicines and Healthcare, P. 39, Oslo, Norway
12   Roth Johnsen J (2006), Health Systems in Transition: Norway, Volume 8 No. 1, 2006, Page 133

Pharmacy PhX and wholesaler WsX are subsidiaries of holding company HoX. PhX wishes to buy a product, whose maximal pharmacy purchasing (AIP) and distribution (AUP) prices are regulated at NOK 70 and NOK 100. Manufacturer Z sells that product at NOK 60 to both wholesalers. PhX and PhY have marginal costs of NOK 20 on each box they sell to patients. WsX and WsY have marginal costs of NOK 5 on every box that they ship to a Norwegian pharmacy. Neither pharmacies nor wholesalers have fixed costs. Both wholesalers supply their own pharmacists at AIP. If PhX buys from WsX, HoX generates total profits of NOK 15 per unit sold. The net profit margin is 33% for PhX, 50% for WsX and 37.5% for HoX. Alternatively, PhX could also buy from WsY. When selling to non-affiliated pharmacists HoY sets the official list price of NOK 70 on which discounts are granted. PhX is requested to pass 50% of any discount received to the public health insurance. From the perspective of HoX the question will be: "What discount will WsY have to offer to make it more attractive to buy from WsY than in-house from WsX?". Above, we have seen that the net margin to Holding company X is 37.5% if wholesaler X is entrusted to buy the product from the manufacturer and sell it to PhX at a price of NOK 70 (AIP). By buying from WsY at a price of NOK 70 and selling to the patient at NOK 100, PhX and HoX attain a net margin of 33% only. PhX has marginal distribution costs of NOK 20 PhX. The difference between the purchasing and the distribution price needs to be NOK 32 to enable PhX to attain a net margin of 37.5% or NOK 12. 37.5% is the net margin that HoX attains when PhX buys from WhX. The minimal discount that HoY needs to offer to PhX so that HoX can reach that threshold is NOK 4. That discount is then split equally between pharmacist X and the national insurance system. HoY would then be operating at a gross margin of NOK 6 and a net margin of NOK 1 or 20%, which is less than the 37.5% that he can attain by selling the drug through his affiliated pharmacy. The optimal strategy for a holding company is therefore to ensure that wholesalers supply their affiliated pharmacies at the official pharmacy purchasing price (AIP).

The flow of pharmaceuticals from the manufacturer to the consumer is illustrated in Figure 2.1. The figure shows that Apotek 1, the Norwegian pharmacy chain of the Phoenix Group, holds a market share of 34.6% on the end consumer market. Phoenix's market share on the wholesale market is almost identical, namely 34.3%. Alliance-Apoteke holds a market share of 18.4% on the end consumer market. Its parent company Unichem holds a share of 20.1% on the wholesale market. The combined shares of Vittus Ditt Apotek (owned by NMD) and Norway's hospital pharmacies are very comparable to the NMD's market share on the wholesale market. We may recall that NMD used to have a monopoly on supplying hospital pharmacies before the liberalization in 1994. These observations suggest that pharmacists tend to buy from the wholesaler they are affiliated to. We assume that revenues of individual wholesalers are more a function of the number of pharmacies they own, than of the competitiveness of the prices they charge.

We observe that pharmacies will now preferably buy from the wholesaler they are affiliated to. This raises the question of how this affects profit sharing between wholesalers and pharmacists? Moreover, it brings up the question of what this means for consumer savings from parallel trade?

When selling a product to an affiliated pharmacy wholesalers will, whenever possible, charge the official pharmacy purchasing price. The rationale behind doing so is that pharmacies buying at a price which is lower than AIP, are requested to reimburse half of the difference between AIP and the effective purchasing price, to public health insurance. Wholesal-

Figure 2.1 The Norwegian supply chain

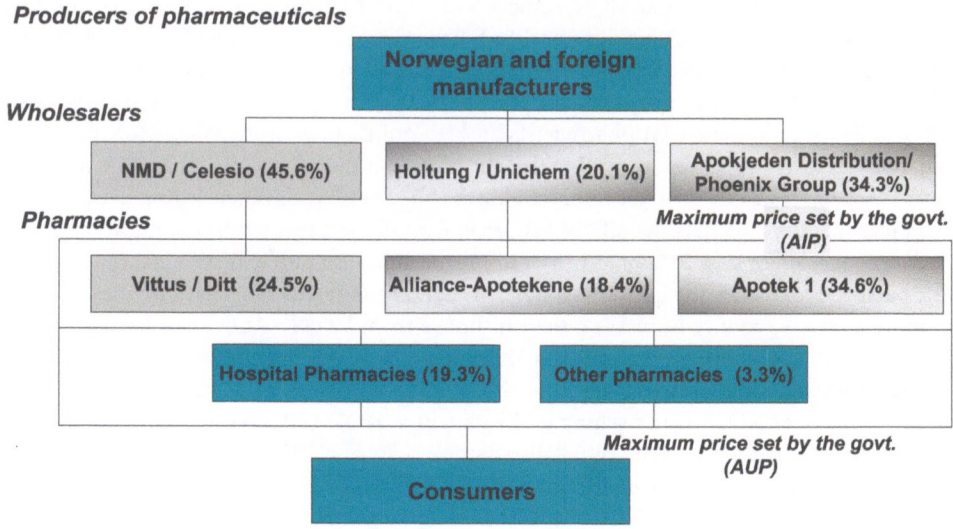

Source: LMI (2007), Facts and Figures 2007: Medicines and Healthcare, P. 38–40, Oslo, Norway

ers, however, can charge AIP irrespective of the list price set by the pharmaceutical company or the parallel trader. Concerning the first question on profit sharing between pharmacists and wholesalers we expect that these are shifted back to the latter party. Moreover, we expect a negative impact on consumer savings from parallel trade. When pharmacies were independent they had incentives to always buy from the wholesaler with the lowest list price. Now, however, the incentive is often to order from the associated wholesaler at the highest possible price, AIP. We expect that incorporating the retail business into the wholesaler chains will lead to increased distribution margins, reduced competition among wholesalers and reduced savings from parallel trade.

A comparison of data on profit sharing between drug manufacturers, wholesalers and pharmacists in the years 2001 and 2005, suggests that wholesaler margins are indeed on the rise, as we predicted. In the year 2005, 9% of the average retail price of a prescription drug (prior to VAT) went to the wholesaler. Four years earlier, in 2001, wholesalers had only been able to cash 4% of the retail price for prescription drugs. That increase went to the expenses of manufacturers and the pharmacists, whose share fell from 76 to 73%, and from 20% to 19% respectively[13].

The relative gap between the pharmacy distribution and the ex-factory price is now higher than when NMD had a monopoly on wholesaling. Seemingly, international wholesalers are more successful in conducting price negotiations than a monopsonist wholesaler,

---

13 Own calculations based on LMI, Facts and Figures 2002 and 2006

who is active in Norway only. Pricing regulations and the structure of the distribution system, however, allow wholesalers to shift these savings around the system[14].

In order to make sure that wholesalers pass their savings to the patient, further measures are needed. The next subchapter presents regulations that are directly targeted on encouraging parallel trade. Later we look at how industry stakeholders respond to these regulations, given the framework presented above.

2.3 How does Norway encourage parallel traded substitution and competition?

2.3.1 Removing technical trade barriers

Pharmaceutical companies are not allowed to sell any product, unless it has been approved by the Norwegian Medicines Agency (NMA). It is NMA's duty to ensure that all pharmaceuticals marketed in Norway are effective and safe. The authorisation process for new products is complicated, costly and time consuming. Pharmaceutical companies who file for a marketing authorisation for new products are requested to submit high amounts of information. The documentation required for a new drugs approval is supposed to tell the drug's whole story, including what happened during the clinical tests, what the ingredients of the drug are, the results of the animal studies, how the drug functions in the body, and how it is manufactured, processed and packaged. This information is needed in order to assess if a product meets NMA's quality and safety requirements. Parallel traded products are, by definition, identical to the locally sourced drug. Asking parallel traders to undergo a full authorisation procedure would be unnecessary and inefficient. The European Commission has set up a directive, quoting that a simplified market authorisation must be given, *"when the product concerned is the same or very similar to a product already authorised for sale in the Member State into which it is to be imported"*[15]. The European Commission leaves it to the EU/EEA member countries own discretion to define what *identical or similar* means. Norway has adopted a flexible view, enabling parallel traders to penetrate the market freely.

a) A relaxed view on pack size deviations
In order to meet patient and government requirements, most products are available in various dosages and pack sizes. The pack size which is registered in Norway may not necessarily be available in any other European country. Most popular pack sizes in Europe are 28 or 30, 56 or 60 and 98 or 100. Drug manufacturers may therefore seek to restrict parallel imports, by arguing that the parallel imported product is not identical or similar to the Norwegian product, if for instance the pack size in Norway is 28 and the one in Spain is 30. Norwegian authorities have always tolerated minor pack size deviations on parallel traded packs[16]. By doing so, they can secure access to parallel traded goods while ensuring that parallel traders do not interfere with the protective cover of a product (e.g. trimming of blisters).

---

14 Interview with Erik A. Stene and Per Olav Kormeset, Oslo, November, 2004

15 European Commission (1982): European Commission Communication AB1 Nr. C 115, 06.05.1982

16 Interview with Erik A. Stene and Per Olav Kormeset, Oslo November 2004

b)   A pragmatic approach to disputes on trade mark violations

Pharmaceutical companies are requested to enclose information leaflets in every box they sell to wholesalers and healthcare providers. These leaflets must provide information on the product, its use and action, side effects and counter indications. Leaflets must be printed in the national language of the country where the product is sold. Some information, such as the brand and non-proprietary name, dosage, pack size and the indication of the product, must also be printed on the *outer box* and the *protective* container. Parallel traders are therefore requested to make some modifications to the products they have bought in Greece or France, before selling them to wholesalers in Norway. These modifications include; replacing the original leaflet with a translated version, and relabeling/overstickering the outer box, so that all relevant information is available in Norwegian. In some cases, parallel traders may have to replace adhesive stickers on the *protective container* of the medicine itself (e.g. bottles, sprays…, etc.). Pharmaceutical companies claim that these modifications constitute an act of trade mark violation. Local authorities, however, argue that these actions are a necessity to make these products marketable in Norway. Rather than restricting trade, Norway has set up clear guidelines, telling parallel traders how to oversticker the original box and when to use new boxes rather than covering the original box with an adhesive sticker. We conclude that technical trade barriers are relatively low in Norway. Pharmaceutical companies are unable to repel parallel imports by practicing incremental product differentiation.

2.3.2   Offering compensation payments to pharmacists who sell lower priced products

Pharmacists are responsible for supplying end consumers with pharmaceuticals and advising them on the use of products or alternatives to the locally sourced brand. Pharmacists have a gate-keeping function when it comes to generics or parallel traded pharmaceuticals. Most European governments are now providing pharmacies with incentives to substitute a cheaper for a more expensive drug. Norwegian pharmacists, for instance, are allowed to keep up to 50% of the price gap between the locally sourced and the parallel traded pharmaceutical. The system induces pharmacists to buy the lowest priced of all parallel traded products and parallel traders to offer competitive prices. In terms of generating savings to the consumers, however, the system is inefficient because half of the savings potential is diverted into the pharmacists' pocket.

2.4   Stakeholder behavioural analysis

The extent, to which a country can benefit from allowing parallel imports, depends on the behaviour of all stakeholders involved in producing, trading, consuming and financing pharmaceuticals. This chapter looks at the principal stakeholders and how they are expected to behave in Norway's regulatory and market environment.

2.4.1   Patient behaviour

Consumer's price sensitivity is a decisive factor in a supplier's pricing behaviour. Parallel traders are likely to undercut their competitors' prices if end consumers are sensitive to small price differences. Patients are more likely to choose a cheaper product if doing so can save them money. Norway caps co-payments of reimbursable benefits to EUR 200 only. Once a patient has reached the co-payment ceiling, he receives the same reimbursement whether he decides to buy the parallel traded or the locally sourced product[17]. Patients suffering from chronic diseases are accountable for the largest share of drug expenditures. Because of the low co-payment cap, such patients have restricted incentives to buy the lowest priced parallel traded product at the pharmacy chain offering the best price. This removes pressure from pharmacy chains to have the lowest priced parallel traded drug available.

2.4.2   Behaviour of independent pharmacies

Pharmacists are allowed to keep 50% of the price difference between the parallel traded and the locally sourced drug. Independent pharmacists have clear incentives to buy from the cheapest supplier.

2.4.3   Behaviour of wholesalers
(with respect to a non-affiliated pharmacy)

In Norway, there are no regulations concerning wholesaler margins. Wholesalers are allowed to charge AIP to pharmacists, no matter what the ex-factory price has been. The only restriction is that parallel traded products have to be cheaper than locally sourced drugs. However, there are no guidelines concerning the minimal price gap between locally sourced and parallel traded drugs. The price gap between the locally sourced and the parallel traded product may, therefore, change between the moment it enters and exits the wholesaler warehouse. The direction of that change depends on the negotiation power of the pharmacist. We have seen that independent pharmacies have incentives to buy from the cheapest supplier, while affiliated pharmacies will generally buy from the incorporated wholesaler at the highest possible price. Independent pharmacies hold a market share of 3% only. Being able to supply independent pharmacies is therefore not vital for a wholesaling company. Independent pharmacies will therefore have difficulties negotiating price reductions with their wholesalers. We should expect wholesalers to retain an important share of the savings they have obtained on their purchases.

---

17 Norway has a reference price system for off-patent drugs. In some cases, patients may therefore be facing additional charges when buying a parallel traded or locally sourced product which is more expensive than the reference price

2.4.4   Behaviour of wholesalers
(with respect to an affiliated pharmacy)

Wholesaler mark ups are free, provided that the parallel traded product is priced below the locally sourced drug. Pharmacists, however, are only entitled to retain 50% of the price difference between the effective price of a drug and AIP. Wholesalers have, therefore, clear incentives to charge the highest possible transfer price to their affiliated wholesalers, both for locally sourced and for parallel traded products.

2.4.5   Behaviour of parallel traders

To start with, it is important to understand that parallel trading companies are run by rational, profit maximising managers. Parallel trading companies will always set the profit maximising price, just as any other firm would do. They will only grant price reductions, if competition or government interventions require them to do so. Norwegian wholesalers have financial incentives to buy from the cheapest supplier. The average price gap between parallel traded and locally sourced drugs shall therefore grow inline with the number of parallel traders. The reason for that is quite simple. In order to be a wholesaler's preferred provider, a parallel trader has to offer significant quantities of a specific product at the lowest price. If several parallel traders are actively marketing the same product, wholesalers will first buy from the cheapest provider. Once the cheapest provider is out of stocks, wholesalers will order from the next more expensive provider. Once all parallel traders have run out of stocks the wholesalers will order from the licensed importer. Because maintaining business relationships with several suppliers involves transaction costs, large parallel traders may nevertheless be able to charge higher prices than small ones.

Rational parallel traders are only inclined to reduce their prices if they are unable to sell their products. Such situations are more likely to occur if cumulated stocks of parallel imported products are close to, at or even above demand. If cumulated stocks are far below domestic demand, wholesalers will readily buy from any importer who is offering a better price than the branded drug manufacturer. Price gaps between locally sourced and parallel traded drugs will then be much smaller.

We recap that the price gap between parallel traded and locally sourced drugs increases with the number of competing parallel traders and the combined market share of all parallel traders. Both conditions are important to ensure effective competition.

2.4.6   Behaviour of pharmaceutical companies

To start with, it is important to understand that subsidiaries of international corporations are not independent in their pricing decision. Instead, they have to set and maintain the price that maximizes global, rather than national profits.

Let us now use a simple example to see how this affects a subsidiary's decision whether or not to repel parallel traded competition by reducing the Norwegian list price. The example is inspired by a model presented by Ganslandt and Maskus in their working paper of the publication *"Parallel imports and the pricing of pharmaceutical products: evidence from the*

European Union"[18]. We have simplified the model to show how a manufacturer's decision whether to deter parallel trade, responds to changes of the market environment. Let us now assume that in Norway, there is one single universal drug X, which is prescribed for all conditions.

- Total expenditures on drug X are capped at NOK 500 m p.a.
- Physicians prescribe X until the whole budget is utilized
- Product X is priced at NOK 500 in Norway and NOK 400 in Greece, where all parallel traded boxes are sourced.
- Transaction costs for creating a new box and importing the product into Norway are NOK 40
- The drug manufacturer can repel parallel traders from the Norwegian market by charging NOK 440 to Norwegian wholesalers, because parallel traded pharmaceuticals have to be cheaper than locally sourced drugs.
- Marginal production costs per unit of X are NOK 250
- If the manufacturer decides to accommodate parallel trade, parallel traders set a price of NOK 460

When parallel traded competition arises, a drug manufacturer will not immediately respond by lowering his prices. Instead, he will observe how market shares of parallel traded products develop. If market shares of parallel imported products are low, the Norwegian subsidiary is better off by giving up a *small proportion* of its home market while maintaining the Norwegian price on the products that can be supplied to Norwegian wholesalers directly. From a certain point, however, the Norwegian subsidiary will be better off by reducing the Norwegian price in order to drive parallel traders out of the market.

Let us now derive a profit function for our Norwegian subsidiary in case that it maintains the old price and allows parallel trade to happen and in case that he decides to deter parallel trade by setting the price in Norway and Greece that makes parallel trade unprofitable.

Given: **Pharmaceutical Budget** $= B_{NOR} = 500.000.000$

$$p_{LS, NOR}^{Allow\ PI} = 500$$

$$p_{GRC} = 400$$

$$mc = 250$$

$$p_{NOR}^{Deny\ PI} = 500$$

$$p_{PI, NOR}^{Allow\ PI} = 460$$

Function 2.1: $\pi_{Norway}^{Allow\ PI} = q_{NOR}(p_{LS, NOR}^{Allow\ PI} - mc) + q_{GRC} \cdot 0$

Function 2.2: $\pi_{Norway}^{Deny\ PI} = (B_{NOR}/p_{NOR}^{Deny\ PI})(p_{NOR}^{Deny\ PI} - mc)$

18 Gansladt M, Maskus K (2001): Parallel Imports of Pharmaceutcials in the European Union, Working Paper No 546, 2001, IUI, Stockholm

Function 2.1 describes the profits for the Norwegian subsidiary from maintaining the official list price (NOK 500). The higher the market share of parallel traded drugs, the lower the profits for the Norwegian subsidiary. Function 2.2 describes the profits for the Norwegian subsidiary from lowering the official list price. Norwegian profits are a function of the pharmacy budget (B_{NO}) and the "uniform" price $p_{NOR}^{Deny\ PI}$. By equating Function 2.1 and 2.2 we find that the Norwegian subsidiary would seek to adapt its price whenever market shares of parallel imported products are higher than 13.6%.

What matters, however, are not Norwegian sales and profits but global sales and profits. Function 2.1 neglects that parallel imported drugs contribute to the drug manufacturer's profits too. We adapt the profit function of the Norwegian subsidiary to take account of products which are imported from Greece.

Function 2.3 describes the budget constraint for pharmaceuticals X in Norway. Function 2.4 describes the profits for the Norwegian subsidiary if the corporation decides to accommodate parallel trade. Parallel imported products which were originally sold to Greek wholesalers are now included in the Norwegian profit function. It shows that Norwegian profits are a negative function of the parallel import penetration in Norway.

Function 2.3: $\quad B_{NO} = q_{NO} \cdot p_{NOR}^{Allow\ PI} + q_{GRC} \cdot p_{GRC}$

Function 2.4: $\quad \pi_{Corporation}^{Allow\ PI} = q_{NOR} \left(p_{NOR}^{Allow\ PI} - mc \right) + q_{GRC} \left(p_{GRC} - mc \right)$

By processing Functions 2.2 through 2.4, we find that the drug manufacturer should charge the market segmentation price whenever market shares of parallel imported pharmaceuticals are lower than 39.2%. In the year 2004, market penetration of parallel traded pharmaceuticals was lower than that for 22 of the 25 top selling pharmaceuticals. When using our model as a reference for a pharmaceutical company's decision making, we find that because market shares of most parallel traded products are only moderate, pharmaceutical companies will often choose to accommodate parallel trade rather than deterring it.

2.4.7 Comments on the behaviour
of industry stakeholders in Norway

Some of the conclusions from above may be difficult to comprehend. We shall therefore spend some more time discussing them.

a) Why would wholesalers be able to abuse
their purchasing power despite competition?

Wholesaler mark-ups have more than doubled since 2001. Pharmacy mark-ups have risen too, though to a smaller extent. Wholesalers have therefore been able to increase their share on the overall distribution mark-up. Interviews with industry representatives[19] suggest that

---

19 Erik A. Stene and Per Olav Kormeset, Oslo November 2004

wholesalers are now more successful in retaining price reductions they have received from their suppliers. The questions of course are: why have wholesaler margins grown and why are they able to shift these savings around the system, despite the competition on the wholesaler market?

The answer is quite simple: by owning their customers. Earlier in this chapter we have shown why wholesalers can generally generate higher returns when supplying their own, rather than non-affiliated pharmacies. Before the liberalization of the retail market, most pharmacies were connected to a centralized purchasing system, which allowed them to always order from the cheapest supplier of a specific product. Wholesalers were therefore under pressure to offer competitive prices. Today, each wholesaler in Norway owns and controls an impressive percentage of the country's pharmacies. Selling discounted pharmaceuticals is no longer a necessity to stay in business. We conclude that distribution margins are on the rise because of lack of competition, not despite competition.

b) Why would parallel traders or pharmaceutical companies reduce their prices if these price cuts are not to the benefit of the end consumer?

Both parallel traders and drug manufacturers are profit driven entrepreneurial entities. An important share of their responsibility is to the investors. Pricing decisions are therefore based on commercial, rather than political terms. It is certainly a parallel traders' right not to accept a wholesaler's conditions. Wholesalers may then simply respond by terminating their business relationship with that parallel trader. Wholesalers do not depend on parallel traders to stay in business. Parallel traders, however, are highly dependent on wholesalers. In the short run pharmaceutical companies and parallel traders have no other choice than accepting the wholesalers' terms.

c) Why do parallel traders not sell to pharmacies and hospitals directly?

In Norway, it requires a wholesaler license to sell pharmaceuticals to pharmacies and hospitals. So far only three wholesaler licenses have been granted. Neither parallel traders nor pharmaceutical companies have any other choice than doing business with wholesalers.

2.5 Parallel trade in Norway an empirical view

2.5.1 Trade volumes

Before Norway entered the European Economic Area in 1994, parallel imports of pharmaceuticals were not permitted. In the first year of its membership Norway allowed parallel imports of non-patented drugs. Parallel imports of patented pharmaceuticals became legal in 1995[20]. The high price level and financial incentives to the pharmacist allowed parallel importers to penetrate the market quickly. By the year 2000, parallel traded pharmaceuticals had acquired a market share of 7.7%, compared to 0.2% in 1995[21]. The introduction of a new

---

20 Bouvy F (2003) Overview of pricing and reimbursement measures taken since January 1993, Working Document, EFPIA, Brussels

21 LMI (2007), Facts and Figures 2007: Medicines and Healthcare, P. 39, Oslo, Norway

benchmarking system in the year 2000, has forced pharmaceutical companies to reduce their prices significantly. By the year 2005, the medicine price index had fallen by 12%, compared to the level in 1999. Despite these price cuts, market shares of parallel traded drugs have only eased back temporarily. In the year 2005, market shares were back at 6.9%, up from 5.1% in 2002. Our research on 25 top selling pharmaceuticals reveals that the average parallel traded pharmaceutical was priced 3% below the locally sourced drug between October 2003 and September 2004. Parallel imported drugs have helped to cut overall drug expenditures by 0.2%. These market shares and price advantages lag far behind European average.

Table 2.1 illustrates how sales of locally sourced and parallel traded drugs developed between 1995 and 2004. Highest growth rates were obviously recorded in the time stretch between 1995 and 2001. Sales and market shares eased back sharply in 2001. Significant price cuts on branded products and the reorganization of the distribution chain had forced parallel traders to (temporarily) withdraw some of their products from the market. In the year 2005, market shares were back at 6.9%.

Table 2.1 Sales of locally sourced and parallel traded pharmaceuticals in Norway (pharmacy distribution prices)

Year	1995	1998	1999	2000	2001	2002	2003	2004
Locally sourced drugs, sales in m NOK	7577	9833	10700	11400	12700	14200	14600	15600
Parallel imports, market share	0.20%	7.0%	6.6%	7.7%	5.1%	6.3%	6.6%	6.3%
Parallel imports, sales in m NOK	15	688	706	878	648	895	963	982

	CAGR 95–04		CAGR 99–04		CAGR 00–04		CAGR 01–04	
Locally sourced drugs	8.3%		7.8%		8.5%		7.0%	
Parallel imported drugs	58.9%		6.8%		2.8%		14.9%	

Source: Own calculations, based on Facts and Figures 2005, LMI, Oslo

2.5.2 Price advantages of parallel imported drugs

a) Description of the data sample used for the calculation of savings from parallel trade

For our evaluation we have selected twenty-six of the top selling products in Norway[22]. Seven of these products are facing generic competition. For seventeen, a parallel imported

---

[22] Sales and Pricing Database for the 25 products provided by Farmastat, a unit of LMI, the Norwegian Association of Pharmaceutical Manufacturers, Sales and Revenue figures cover the time period between October 1st, 2003 and September 30th, 2004

version is available. In the twelve month period between October 2003 and September 2004, these products generated revenues of 2.7 bn NOK at pharmacy purchasing prices, thus accounting for approximately 27% of the 10.1 bn drug market in Norway[23]. Market penetration of parallel imported drugs within our sample is 15.4%, compared to a weighted 6.3% for the total market. That of generics within our sample is 6.4%, compared to a weighted 9.1% for the total market. Our sample covers 66.2% of the market for parallel traded drugs, 19% of the generic market and 25% of the market for locally sourced & branded drugs. Table 2.2 provides an overview of the 26 products which are included in our survey. Products are ordered by therapeutic subgroup, generic and brand name. The last two columns in the upper half of the table indicate whether a product is exposed to generic or parallel traded competition. The lower quarter of Table 2.2 provides an overview of revenues generated by locally sourced and parallel traded brands and generics in the period between October 2003 and September 2004. It repeats the figures presented earlier in this paragraph.

b) Description of the methodology used for the calculation of savings
Our data sample provides detailed information on a products' property including its non proprietary name and brand name, dosage, pack size and suppliers' classification (locally sourced brand, parallel traded brand, generic). For each product, Farmastat provided information on the maximal pharmacy purchasing price (AIP, as published by NMA), the number of units sold and total revenues at pharmacy purchasing prices. Sales information refers to the full time period between October 2003 and September 2004.

The average sales price per unit sold is calculated by dividing total revenues by the number of packs sold during that twelve month period. When comparing the average prices of locally sourced and parallel traded brands, we find that in some cases the parallel traded version was more expensive than the locally sourced pack for the same time period, dosage form and pack size. Legally parallel traded products have to be cheaper than their locally sourced rival. If the average price for parallel traded drugs sold is higher than the average price for the locally sourced drug we can conclude that the price of the locally sourced product has fallen during the observation period. In Norway prescription drugs are subject to price volume contracts. These contracts force pharmaceutical companies to grant substantial price reductions if prescription volumes exceed pre-defined targets. It is, therefore, common that a locally sourced pharmaceutical starts selling at a price $AIP = \alpha$ in January before being adjusted to $AIP = \alpha - \beta$ during the year. If $AIP = \alpha - \beta$ is lower than the price charged by the parallel trader who decides to quit selling that product for the remainder of the year, it is possible that over a twelve month period, locally sourced products are cheaper than their parallel traded competitors.

In order to avoid any misinterpretation we remove all products with incoherent pricing patterns from our sample. Sales of parallel traded packs which are represented in our final sample accounted for NOK 233 m, representing 37% of total PI sales in 2003/2004[24].

---

23 Assuming that ¼ of 2003 sales were generated between Oct 2003 and Dec 2004 and ¾ of 2004 sales between Jan 2004 and Sep 2004

24 Oct 2003– Sep2004

Table 2.2 Information on the competitive situation and revenues of the 26 products selected for Norway

ATC4 class	ATC Code	Generic name	Brand name	Exposed to PI	Exposed to generics
Proton Pump Inhibitors	A02BC05	Esomperazole	Nexium	YES	NO
	A02BC01	Omeprazole	Losec	YES	YES
	A02BC03	Lanzoprazole	Lanzo	YES	NO
Cholesterol Lowering Agents	C10AA05	Atrovastatine	Lipitor	YES	NO
	C10AA01	Simvastatin	Zocor	YES	YES
	C10AA03	Pravastatin	Pravachol	YES	YES
Beta Blocking Ag.	C08CA01	Amolidipine	Norvasc	YES	YES
Ca. Channel Bl.	C07AB02	Metoprolol	Selo-Zok	YES	YES
ACE II Inhibitors	C09CA01	Losartan	Cozaar	NO	NO
	C09CA03	Valsartan	Diovan	NO	NO
Tetracycline	J01FA10	Clarithromycin	Klacid	NO	YES
	J01FA09	Azithromycin	Zythromax	NO	NO
Selective Immunosuppressive	L04AA01	Ciclosporin	Sandimmun	YES	NO
	L04AA05	Tacrolimus	Prograf	YES	NO
	L04AA6	Mycophenolic a.	Cellcept	YES	NO
Bisphosphonats	M05BA04	Alendronic acid	Fosamax	NO	NO
Coxibs	M01AH01	Rofecoxib	Vioxx	YES	NO
Antipsychotics	N05AH03	Olezapine	Zyprexa	YES	NO
	N05AX08	Risperidone	Risperdal	YES	NO
Antidepressiva	N06AB04	Citalopram	Cipramil	NO	YES
	N06AB06	Sertraline	Zoloft	YES	NO
	N06AX16	Venlafaxin	Efexor	NO	YES
Anti-Dementiva	N06DA02	Donepezil	Aricept	YES	NO
Ardeneric Inhalants	R03AK06	Salmeterol	Seretide	YES	NO
	R03AK07	Formoterol	Symbicort	YES	NO
Glucocorticoids	R03BA02	Budesonide	Pulmicort	YES	NO
	Total	Branded locally sourced	PI	Generic	
Sales total market ('000 NOK)	10 071 500	8 524 200	634 000	913 300	
% of total market	100%	84.6%	6.3%	9.1%	
Sales sample ('000 NOK)	2 724 594	2 131 456	419 679	173 459	
% of Sample	100%	78.2%	15.4%	6.4%	
% of relative market	27.1%	25.0%	66.2%	19.0%	

c)   Average price advantages of parallel imported products and savings resulting for the NHS

In the twelve month period between October 2003 and September 2004, parallel traded drugs were priced 3% below the locally sourced rival[25]. With a total turnover of NOK 233 m, parallel imported drugs which are included in our sample generated savings of NOK 7.3 m at pharmacy purchasing prices. Sales of all parallel traded drugs in Norway amounted to NOK 634 m. Assuming that the 3% price difference between locally sourced and parallel traded drugs is representative for the entire market, the latter product group would have generated savings of NOK 19.5 m at pharmacy purchasing prices. What matters to the consumer, however, are the savings at *pharmacy distribution* prices. In the years 2003/2004 the ratio between pharmacy purchasing and distribution prices was 0.658. At pharmacy distribution prices, parallel traded products would therefore have generated sales of NOK 964 m and savings of NOK 30.1 m. Because pharmacies are entitled to keep half of the price difference between the parallel traded and the locally sourced drug, effective savings broke down to NOK 15.1 m or NOK 3.3 m per capita. In Euro terms, savings would have totalled to EUR 1.8 m or EUR 0.40 per capita. These figures are summarized in Table 2.3

Table 2.3 Savings from parallel trade in Norway

	Revenue PI	Revenue PI at prices of locally sourced drugs	Savings
Sample, pharmacy purchasing prices (m NOK)	232.7	240.0	7.3
Total market, pharmacy purchasing prices (m NOK)	634.0	653.8	19.8
Total market, pharmacy distribution prices (m NOK)	963.5	993.6	15.1
Total market, pharmacy distribution prices (m EUR)	115.0	118.6	1.8
Total market per capita pharmacy distribution prices (NOK)	211.4	218	3.30

Source: Own calculations based on Farmastat sales database and Facts and Figures 2005, LMI, 2005

d)   Price advantages and savings from individual products

In the year 2004, savings from parallel traded drugs in Norway accounted for 0.2% of total drug expenditures. Table 2.4 shows that price advantages of parallel imported drugs vary considerably. The three most attractively priced products generated 42.3% of all savings even though only accounting for 9.5% of all sales. The three least attractively priced products generated 9.8% of all savings while representing 48.1% of all sales. Market penetration of parallel imported products was 4.9% for the three products where price advantages

---

25 Weighted for sales

Table 2.4 Price advantages and savings from parallel trade in Norway, numbers at million NOK

	Price advantages (%)	% of total sales	% of total savings	Sales	Sales at prices of locally sourced drugs	Savings
Three most attractively priced	12.2%	9.5%	42.3%	22.2	25.3	3.1
Rest	3.4%	42.4%	47.9%	98.6	102.1	3.5
Three least attractively priced	0.6%	48.1%	9.8%	111.9	112.6	0.7
TOTAL	3.0%	100%	100%	232.7	240.0	7.3

Source: Own calculations based on Farmastat sales database and Facts and Figures 2005, LMI, 2005

were highest compared to 28% for the three products where price advantages were lowest. There is, however, no correlation (neither positive nor negative) between price advantage and market penetration.

Whilst knowing that pharmacies are compensated for selling a cheaper drug, one may be surprised that parallel imported products which are priced closest to the locally sourced drug, sell that well in Norway. The paradox, however, is reflected in the ownership structure of the Norwegian retail market. Wholesalers, as we know, are bound to the maximum pharmacy purchasing price. We shall, therefore, conclude that the three parallel traded products in question do not sell well because they were expensive in procurement, but more because they allowed Norwegian wholesalers to retain the highest margins.

2.6   Summary and proposals for policy reforms

Norway is the European country with the lowest relative savings from parallel trade. Even though parallel importers are under pressure to compete with prices, consumers do not benefit from this competition. The reason being, that wholesalers are able to shift received price reductions around the system. We have, therefore, identified three proposals for future policy reforms that would lead to an improvement of the current parallel trade situation.

a)   Disjunction of the wholesale and the pharmacy system
The structure of the drug distribution system is currently the most important reason why patients hardly benefit from parallel trade. The ownership of the pharmacy system allows wholesalers to shift most of the savings they achieved on procurement around the system. The disjunction of the wholesale and the pharmacy system is, therefore, an ultimate requirement for competition that will be to the benefit of the consumer.

b)   Reform of the pharmacy compensation system
The current legislation allows pharmacists in Norway to retain up to 50% of the price difference between the locally sourced and the parallel traded/generic drug. Compensating pharmacists for dispensing a lower priced product is inefficient because half of the potential

savings are lost to the middlemen. Rather than "bribing" pharmacists to act cost-responsibly, Norway should enforce generic competition, for example, by setting the directive that pharmacists always dispense the cheapest of all chemically identical products.

c)   Reform of the patient reimbursement system:

Under the current reimbursement system, the chronically ill have very few incentives to switch to a lower priced product, especially if the product is still under patent protection. By chopping reimbursement to the price of the cheapest of all chemically identical products, Norway would increase the cost awareness of its patients. This would maintain the pressure on parallel traders to offer competitive prices and drive savings to the consumer up. Moreover it would increase demand for lower priced products, thus easing market access to parallel traders and generic companies.

3

Parallel trade of pharmaceutical drugs in Denmark

3.1 Summary

In Denmark, wholesalers started selling parallel traded drugs to hospitals in 1992, responding to demand for lower priced products. After the government had implemented a series of health policy reforms, including a law that required pharmacists to dispense parallel traded products, the respective sales and market shares picked up markedly. By the third quarter of the 1990s, parallel import penetration had grown to approximately 10% where it stabilized despite a significant, government induced, reduction of average prices on locally sourced brands starting in 1999.

Based on a sample of 47 top selling drugs, we have estimated relative price advantages of and savings from parallel traded drugs for the time period between January 2002 and July 2004. In that period, the average parallel traded pack was priced 7.8% below the locally sourced drug. Savings per head and per annum accounted for 3.5 EUR or 0.9% of total drug expenditures. We find that the average price difference between the parallel traded and the locally sourced drug is higher if the latter is exposed to generic competition too (17.3%) compared to the situation when it is not (5.3%). Moreover we find evidence that the price difference between the locally sourced and the parallel traded drug grows inline with the number of parallel traders who are selling the same product at the same time.

3.2 The Danish Healthcare System

3.2.1 Organization

Healthcare in Denmark is mainly funded through taxation, by the local governments. The central government is responsible for defining and coordinating healthcare goals, while counties and municipalities are financing and providing almost all healthcare for their citizens. The main sources of finance are county and municipal taxes. Other sources include out-of pocket payments and voluntary health insurance to cover part of these out of pocket payments[26].

---

26 Vallgårda S. et al. (2001), Healthcare Systems in Transition: Denmark

In Denmark general practitioners have a gate-keeper function and are responsible for providing basic healthcare services for the population. Only authorised and licensed physicians can have their services reimbursed by the National Insurance System. The general practitioners compensation model has two elements:
1. A per capita payment for every registered patient
2. Fee for service reimbursement for each consultation, with different rates for different types of consultations

Fixed per capita payments represent 30%–50% of a physicians' income. Activity based compensations and co-payments account for the rest[27]. The combination of capitation and fee for service payments encourages physicians to cure patients themselves, rather than just referring them to clinics. Moreover, it prevents them from providing unnecessary services. Physicians need to have a license in order to work as general practitioners. The threat of having their license removed provides incentives to act inline with the authorities' directives.

Hospitals in Denmark are managed and financed by municipalities. They control the number of hospital beds, the amount of personnel and any investments in new technologies that hospitals make. Most hospitals receive global budgets for their inpatient activities. These budgets are based on past performance and modified at the margin to account for new activities, changes in tasks and areas of specific need[28]. Global budgets are an effective cost containment tool in stationary care. However, they limit a hospitals' flexibility to respond to patient needs and do not reward efficiency.

We conclude that the government controls in- and out-patient expenditures through: the limitation of the number and the selection of healthcare professionals in primary care, the gate keeping function of general practitioners and the ownership and control of the hospital market.

Drug manufacturers and parallel traders are privately run, *profit maximizing* businesses. The government cannot dictate to drug manufacturers which product shall be developed. Neither can it tell parallel traders which drugs to offer. They have no direct influence on the availability or the prices of parallel traded pharmaceuticals. Instead, the government has to influence the behaviour of those stakeholders who are prescribing, distributing and buying parallel traded pharmaceuticals. Inducing parallel traders to behave in a desired way is, therefore, more difficult than inducing government controlled hospitals to do the same thing. In the next subchapters we will look at how successful the government is in influencing stakeholder's behaviour.

3.2.2 Reimbursement of pharmaceuticals

Pharmaceuticals in Denmark are divided in two categories: over the counter and prescription drugs. Over the counter drugs are not eligible for reimbursement by the National Insurance System, prescription drugs are. Expenditure on prescription drugs is subject to

27 Vallgårda S. et al. (2001), Healthcare Systems in Transition: Denmark, Vol. 8, Nr. 7
28 Vallgårda S. et al. (2001), Healthcare Systems in Transition: Denmark, Vol. 8, Nr. 7

different levels of patient co-payment. The calculation of the reimbursement to patients is based on the total cost of products purchased during the last twelve months. No subsidy is granted as long as total costs do not exceed DKK 500. If total costs are higher, patients are reimbursed 50 percent of the portion exceeding DKK 500 but less than DKK 1 200, 75 percent of the portion exceeding DKK 1 200 but less than DKK 2 800, 85 percent of the portion exceeding DKK 2 800 but less than DKK 3 600 and 100 percent of total cost exceeding DKK 3 600.

A patient, with an annual consumption of DKK 3 600 (EUR 485), will therefore endure costs of DKK 1 370[29]. In 2004, out of pocket payments accounted for 39.9% of total expenditures on prescription drugs[30]. The average patient has, therefore, strong financial incentives to switch to lower priced products. Because co-payments on pharmaceuticals in Denmark are higher than in any other western European country, we can expect Danish patients to be more sensitive towards drug prices than other Europeans.

3.2.3 The price setting process for pharmaceuticals

The Danish Medicines Agency (Lægemiddelstyrelsen/DKMA) is the national regulatory authority for new and existing medicines. It regulates reimbursement prices and trade conditions of pharmaceuticals. Other responsibilities include: supervision, production, trials and marketing and the evaluation and authorisation of new medicines.

Unlike most European agencies, DKMA does not explicitly regulate ex-factory, pharmacy purchasing or distribution prices. Instead it sets a maximal reimbursement price. Calculation of this price is based on the average pharmacy purchasing price in all EU/EEA countries except Greece, Luxemburg, Portugal and Spain. Pharmaceutical companies are allowed to charge a higher than the maximal reimbursement price. If they do so, patients have to pay the full difference out of their own pocket[31]. Drug manufacturers and parallel traders are requested to submit pricing information on their products at launch and inform the agency on any changes. Every fortnight DKMA publishes a list with binding pharmacy purchasing and distribution prices for all products. DKMA compiles that list based on the information which has been provided by the marketing authorisation holders. Retailer margins are a positive function of the pharmacy distribution price. Individual pharmacists have incentives to dispense higher priced products. Ex factory prices, and – implicitly – wholesaler margins are negotiated between wholesalers and pharmaceutical companies or parallel traders. They are generally a positive function of the pharmacy distribution price. With no further measures in place, we should therefore expect pharmacies and wholesalers to be reluctant towards the thought of dispensing lower priced medicines. The next subsection looks at how Denmark is dealing with that issue and how the respective measures are affecting sales and prices of parallel traded medicines.

---

29 Vallgårda S. et al. (2001), Healthcare Systems in Transition: Denmark, Vol. 8, Nr. 7, Page 30

30 EFPIA (2006), The Pharmaceutical Industry in Figures, Page 37, Brussels

31 Bouvy F. (2003) Overview of pricing and reimbursement measures taken since January 1993, Working Document, EFPIA, Brussels

3.2.4   The distribution chain of pharmaceuticals in Denmark

a)   Wholesalers

Denmark has three wholesalers distributing drugs to pharmacies within the country. Unlike in Norway, pharmaceutical companies and parallel traders are allowed to supply pharmacists directly. Wholesaling companies, however, are generally more efficient in supplying pharmacies, due to their ability to make use of economies of scale. The hospital market is handled by AMGROS, a publicly owned distribution company. AMGROS buys from wholesalers, pharmaceutical companies and parallel traders.

National regulations require wholesalers to charge the official list price – as published by DKMA – to all pharmacies in Denmark. However, they are entitled to offer cost-related discounts if they have, for instance obtained a price reduction from their supplier or managed to reduce their operating expenses. If discounts were prohibited, wholesalers would have few incentives to increase their efficiency or to pass obtained price reductions to the pharmacists. Moreover, the provision allowing pharmaceutical companies, parallel traders and wholesalers to offer cost related discounts eases market access to parallel traders and increases competition among wholesalers. Promotional discounts, however, remain illegal. In practice it may be difficult for a court to prove that the discount a parallel trader offers to wholesaler X is purely promotional and not cost related[32].

b) Pharmacists

Pharmaceuticals in Denmark are distributed by *privately owned* pharmacies. At present, legal entities are not allowed to own or run pharmacies. There are consequently no pharmacy chains in Denmark. The ministry of health decides on the number and geographical location of pharmacies. Combined gross profits off all pharmacies in Denmark are fixed every two years on the basis of current figures and forecasts. Every fortnight the Danish Medicine Agency publishes binding pharmacy purchasing and distribution prices for every product marketed in Denmark[33]. Pharmacy mark-ups, which are a positive function of ex-factory prices, are set in a way that allows pharmacists to attain their profit margins. Individual pharmacists can therefore increase their profits and salaries by dispensing more expensive products.

A provision passed in 2001, allows pharmacists to retain up to 50% of any discount they receive from their suppliers[34]. When having the choice between two parallel traded products with the same list price, pharmacists will select the one which is more heavily discounted.

---

32   Interview with Jørgen Clausen, Copenhagen, June 4th, 2004

33   Accessible at: http://www.laegemiddelstyrelsen.dk/1024/visLSArtikel.asp?artikelID=1431

34   Bouvy F (2003) Overview of pricing and reimbursement measures taken since January 1993, Working Document, EFPIA, Brussels

3.3 How does Denmark encourage parallel traded substitution and competition?

3.3.1 Removing technical trade barriers

According to Articles 28/29 of the EC treaty, quantitative restrictions on imports/exports between Member States and all measures having equivalent effect, shall be prohibited. According to Article 30, the provisions of Articles 28 and 29 shall not preclude prohibitions or restrictions [...] justified on grounds of [...] public security; the *protection of health* and life of humans, [...] or the *protection of industrial and commercial property*[35]. Such prohibitions or restrictions shall not, however, constitute a means of arbitrary discrimination or a disguised restriction of trade between Member States.

Legitimate patient safety concerns would allow authorities to deny marketing authorisation for a specific product. It would, for instance, be legitimate to deny market authorisation for a parallel traded drug which has different storage and handling requirements than the locally sourced product. We can think of a situation where the two formulations of a drug are sold to patients in Greece and Denmark. The old formulation, which is still for sale in Greece, must be stored in a fridge. The new formulation, for sale in Denmark, can be kept at room temperature. It is obvious, that allowing parallel traders to sell the Greek formulation to Danish patients could endanger lives.

a)   Tolerance towards different presentation forms and formulations
In order to meet patient needs, identical products may come along in different forms. The formulation of a product may influence its bioavailability or pharmacokinetics. In other cases, however, the formulation may have no significant impact on the way a product works in the body. Coated pills, for instance, are easier to swallow or better in taste than non-coated pills. The coating substance is generally designed to have no impact on the bioavailability of the product. Depending on local needs, pharmaceutical companies may, therefore, sell either or both versions of the same drug. Our evaluation shows that DKMA generally makes no difference between coated and non-coated forms, meaning that parallel traders are able to import the coated formulation of a drug, even if it is not distributed by the property right holder in Denmark. We find that the DKMA has a pragmatic view on product safety issues. Drug manufacturers are unable to prevent parallel trade from happening by practicing marginal product differentiation.

b)   Tolerance towards pack size deviations
All products, which are subsidised by public health insurance, are published on a reimbursement list. This list sorts products by non-proprietary name, brand name, form, pack size and dosage. Because of different regulatory requirements or changing marketing strategies, pack sizes for identical products are often not the same in Denmark and other European countries. In order to facilitate parallel trade, Danish authorities have set the standard that paral-

---

35   Treaty establishing the European Community, Official Journal C 325 of 24 December 2002, European Union

lel trade applications shall be granted if the pack size deviation between the foreign and the domestic pack is no higher than 10% for prescription and 25% for OTC drugs[36].

c)   Clear rules concerning the use of the property right holder's brand

When applying for a marketing-authorisation, parallel traders need to make suggestions to DKMA concerning the design of the box and the leaflet they wish to use for their product. Once a product has been approved by DKMA, it is up to the drug manufacturer to decide whether or not to sue the parallel trader for breach of property rights. Doing so has, for a long time, been a common strategy used by pharmaceutical companies, not necessarily because they were expecting to win the lawsuit, but more because they intended to drive the parallel traders' costs up, thus setting disincentives to engage in parallel trade in the first place[37]. These legal disputes have produced a considerable amount of case law describing what parallel traders may and may not do.

Today there is a general consensus, that parallel traders should use adhesive stickers, to cover the property right holder's box. The stickers need to cover all six sides of the box, the company emblem and the name of the proprietor as well as the trade-mark emblem of the product. Parallel traders should use white stickers and refrain from creating own brand emblems for different products. If the foreign and the domestic names are different, parallel traders should use the non-proprietary name. If they are similar (e.g. Aspirin/Aspirine), the foreign brand name may be used. If the foreign and the domestic brand name are identical, the parallel trader may use that brand name.

The repackaging requirements appear strict, at first sight. This, however, does not mean that parallel traders are unable to create their own brand. In practice, coloured company emblems appear on the boxes of most parallel traded goods. Paranova, the second player uses white stickers with two coloured stripes on either edge of the box. The company emblem and name is prominently placed on the lower left corner on the face side and on the flaps. Orifarm, the market leader uses white stickers and the company logo without any additional graphical elements[38]. Parallel importers in Scandinavia are highly professional and their products look neat and clean.

d)   Conclusions

Product related entry hurdles have not been a big issue in Denmark's recent parallel trade history. The assessment, whether a parallel import license can be granted to a product is solely based on therapeutic equivalence or bioequivalence. A license is granted, whenever both versions produce essentially the same biological availability of the active substance in the body when given in the same quantity. Trimming of blisters is not tolerated for product safety and traceability reasons.

Parallel traders are, nevertheless, allowed to import packs with sizes which are unavailable in Denmark. Drug manufacturers are consequently unable to segment markets by selling smaller or larger packs to consumers in Denmark. A relaxed view on property rights and a pragmatic approach on patient safety issues allows parallel traders unrestricted access to the Danish drug market.

---

36   Interview with Bøgh-Sørensen et al., Orifarm A/S, Odense, 06.06.2004

37   Interview with Bøgh-Sørensen et al. Orifarm A/S, 06.05.2004, Odense, Denmark

38   Interview with Bøgh-Sørensen H. et al., Orifarm A/S, 06.05.2004, Odense, Denmark

3.3.2 Providing financial incentives to patients to buy lower priced products

The maximal reimbursement price for a pharmaceutical in Denmark is equal to the lower of the following two: the average European price or the lowest priced product within the Danish reference basket[39].

The reference basket includes all products with the same active ingredient, dosage and pack size. If alternatives to the locally sourced brand are available, reimbursement is capped to the price of the cheapest parallel traded (or generic) drug, provided that it is priced below the European average price. In Denmark, prices of all products are freely available in the internet and upon request at DKMA. Patients are therefore able to check for lower priced alternatives and request a cheaper parallel traded or generic product from their pharmacist. Informed and price sensitive end consumers are an important condition for price competition among parallel traders.

3.3.3 Giving directives to pharmacists to dispense lower priced products

Pharmacies in Denmark are requested to dispense the parallel traded version of a drug if the locally sourced drug is priced at or below 100 and the price gap between both versions exceeds 5 DKK. If the product is priced between 100 and 400 DKK, pharmacists are requested to dispense the parallel traded product if the gap exceeds 5%. If the product is priced above 400 DKK, pharmacists are requested to dispense the parallel traded product if the price gap exceeds 20 DKK[40].

If the price difference between the parallel traded and the locally sourced product is lower than that, pharmacists are requested to inform the patient about the availability and the price of that product. It is then up to the patient to decide which product to buy. If several parallel traded products are available, pharmacists are requested to dispense the cheapest one. Giving directives to pharmacists to always dispense the cheapest of all interchangeable products is an effective measure to induce competition among parallel traders. We shall therefore expect price gaps between parallel traded and locally sourced products to be higher than in Norway.

3.3.4 Monitoring by municipal authorities and the Ministry of Health[41]

Municipal authorities have appointed inspectors who are monitoring the pharmacists' procurement and distribution behaviour. The monitoring system, allows them to identify pharmacies that are not complying with the dispensation law. Deviations are strategically

---

39 Bouvy F. (2003) Overview of pricing and reimbursement measures taken since January 1993, Working Document, EFPIA, Brussels

40 Bouvy F (2003) Overview of pricing and reimbursement measures taken since January 1993, Working Document, EFPIA, Brussels

41 Interview with H. Bøgh-Sørensen et al., Orifarm A/S, Odense, 06.06.2004

reported back to the Ministry of Health. The ministry is appointed to bring any faulty pharmacist back on track. In a first step, pharmacists are generally informed that their non-compliance has been detected. Furthermore pharmacists are informed about the consequences that may result (removal of the license) from such misconduct. Talks with parallel traders and representatives of the pharmaceutical industry have shown that the co-operation between parallel traders, wholesalers and the inspectors works well, a matter that facilitates the detection of non-complying pharmacists. Up to date, no pharmacist has lost his license due to non-compliance[42].

3.3.5   The Danish media[42]

Interviews conducted with parallel traders revealed that newspapers and television channels have been reporting names of pharmacists who failed to supply generic or parallel traded substitutes of locally sourced brands if those would have been available. Also, names of physicians who checked the "Substitution Prohibited" box too often were brought to the attention of the public. Fearing bad press and increased scrutiny of government inspectors, most pharmacists and physicians have decided to act inline with the law.

3.4   Stakeholder behaviour analysis

The extent to which a country can benefit from allowing parallel imports depends on the behaviour of all stakeholders involved in producing, trading, consuming and financing pharmaceuticals. This chapter looks at the principal stakeholders and how they're expected to behave in Denmark's regulatory and market environment.

3.4.1   Patient behaviour

The current reimbursement system sets incentives to buy the cheapest available interchangeable product. Interchangeable products are pharmaceuticals with the same active substance, dosage and pharmacokinetics. We shall, therefore, expect Danes to insist on receiving the cheapest of all parallel traded or generic product versions, thus putting pressure on pharmacists to have these drugs available in their outlet.

3.4.2   Pharmacists behaviour

Pharmacists are requested to always dispense the cheapest of all interchangeable products. Compliance with these directives is effectively monitored both by authorities and the media. Non-compliance may result in losing their license. Pharmacists have therefore *vital* incen-

---

42   Interview with H. Bøgh-Sørensen et al., Orifarm A/S, Odense, 06.06.2004

Table 3.1 Pharmacy distribution mark-ups for locally sourced and parallel traded drugs in Denmark

Nexium 40 mg 14pcs	AIP	AUP	Margin	Loss to the pharmacist	Minimal discount for full compensation
Astra Zeneca A/S	162.11	232.7	70.59	0	0
2care4 aps	153.05	220.4	67.35	−3.24	6.48
Orifarm A/S	153.05	220.4	67.35	−3.24	6.48

Source: Own calculations based on DKMA (2006)

tives to comply with these regulations. *Financially* speaking, however, it is unattractive for pharmacists to buy and dispense a lower priced product. Distribution mark-ups are a positive function of the pharmacy purchasing price of a product. Buying a product with a reduced list price results in getting a lower distribution margin.

The Danish law allows wholesalers to offer discounts on the official list price, provided that these discounts are *cost related*. Pharmacies are entitled to keep 50% of any discounts received. The other 50% have to be used to reduce the pharmacy distribution price. If the discount on a parallel traded product is high enough, the pharmacist may, therefore, attain a higher margin than when selling the locally sourced product.

To understand why, let us look at the following example. On October, 28th, 2006 two parallel traded and one locally sourced "Nexium 40 mg, 14 pcs" were on the Danish market. The substitution law requires pharmacists to always dispense the lowest priced of all available products. Providing availability, pharmacists were therefore requested to dispense the parallel imported "Nexium Orifarm" or "Nexium 2care4". The locally sourced product "Nexium AstraZeneca" was priced at DKK 232.7 (Pharmacy Distribution Price). Parallel imported "Nexium Orifarm" and "Nexium 2care4" were both priced at DKK 220.4, 5.6% below the locally sourced product. The pharmacy mark up for a box of "Nexium Astra Zeneca" is DKK 70.59. The pharmacy mark-up for a parallel traded box of "Nexium Orifarm" or "Nexium 2care4" was DKK 67.35. With every parallel traded box he sells, the pharmacist loses DKK 3.24. Whenever the discount on the parallel traded drug is higher than DKK 6.48 it is, financially speaking, more attractive for the pharmacists to buy the parallel traded drug. The pharmacists will buy from the parallel trader who offers the highest discount. These results are summarized in Table 3.1.

We summarize that a pharmacist will always buy and dispense the lowest priced of all interchangeable products which are currently available (locally sourced or parallel traded brand or generic). If the same price is charged by several suppliers and no lower priced alternative is available, pharmacists buy from the one which is offering the highest discount.

3.4.3 Wholesalers' behaviour

The commercial freedom of Danish wholesalers is highly restricted. National regulations require all wholesalers to charge – for a specific product – the same *list price* to all pharmacists.

Binding pharmacy purchasing prices for all pharmaceuticals are published every fortnight by DKMA. Wholesaler purchasing prices are negotiated between wholesalers and pharmaceutical companies or parallel traders. Manufacturers and parallel traders are requested to submit these prices to DKMA and inform the agency of any changes. Wholesaler margins resulting from price negotiations with suppliers are generally a positive function of the ex-factory price. This means that wholesalers prefer to sell more expensive products. A law passed in 1995 requires wholesalers to buy any quantity of parallel traded products that the market is able to absorb. Because pharmacists are requested to always dispense the lowest priced of all interchangeable products, we expect wholesalers to always have that product available in their warehouse.

Just like pharmacies, wholesalers are entitled to receive discounts, provided that these discounts are cost related. Wholesalers are requested to pass these discounts down to the pharmacists and public health insurance. In practice, wholesalers may be able to retain a share of these discounts for their own purposes[43].

3.4.4 Behaviour of parallel traders

So far we have found that all downstream players from the wholesaler to the patient have either incentives or obligations to buy from the lowest priced provider. Pharmacies are requested to dispense the parallel imported product, whenever it is more than 5% cheaper than the locally sourced drug. We shall, therefore, expect parallel traders to use that 5% gap as a reference for their pricing decisions.

A first entrants' best choice is to charge a price which is exactly five percent below that of the locally sourced drug (no less than DKK 5 and no more than DKK 20). If additional parallel traders start selling the same product, competition may force the incumbent parallel trader and any new entrant to reduce the price. In Denmark parallel traders may additionally or alternatively choose to offer a discount.

Promotional discounts are prohibited. However, wholesalers will seek to flexibly adapt their discounts to take account of an individual wholesaler's purchasing power and price elasticity. Overall, parallel traders can generate higher profits by selectively offering discounts (implicit price discrimination) than by applying the same list price for all wholesalers. Reducing the *list price* becomes inevitable if the parallel trader is no longer able to sell his products at the conditions he offers. This is more likely to happen if combined stocks of all parallel traders are close to or above domestic demand.

Market entrants are expected to undercut incumbent prices in order to quickly generate sales and push their product through the supply chain. If combined supplies of all parallel traders remain behind domestic demand, the new importer will align his price to the level of the incumbent suppliers. We summarize that price advantages of parallel traded products grow inline with the number of active competitors and the ratio between supplies of parallel traded pharmaceuticals and domestic demand.

---

43 Interview with J. Clausen, June, 2004

3.4.5　Behaviour of pharmaceutical companies

Danish sales organizations of multinational companies are requested to set the price that maximises corporate profits. The chapter on Norway has shown that from the perspective of the local sales organization, parallel trade is more harmful than from the perspective of the corporation as a whole. For this reason, requests posted by national sales organizations to reduce prices as a response to parallel trade are often rejected by the global headquarters. Denmark's pharmaceutical market is 15% larger in sales than the Norwegian market[44]. Danish prices for top selling pharmaceuticals are 19% above the Norwegian level[45]. We use the example from the last chapter to see how this affects the corporations pricing decision.

- Total expenditures on product X are capped at EUR 51.5 m p.a.
- Physicians prescribe X until the whole budget is utilized
- Product X is priced at EUR 60 in Denmark and EUR 40 in Greece, where all parallel traded boxes are sourced.
- Transaction costs for creating a new box and importing the product into Denmark are EUR 4
- The drug manufacturer can repel parallel traders from the Danish market by charging EUR 44 to Danish wholesalers
- Marginal production costs per unit of X are EUR 25
- If the manufacturer decides to accommodate parallel trade, parallel traders set a price of EUR 55

By inserting these values into Functions 2.1 and 2.2 and equating we find that the Danish marketing authorisation would choke parallel trade by setting a price of EUR 44, whenever market shares of parallel imported products exceed 26%.

From the perspective of the corporation as a whole, however, it is unreasonable to do so before parallel imported products have exceeded a market share of 48.8%. In the year 2004, parallel import penetration was higher than 48.8% for ten out of 48 products which are included in our survey. However, because price cuts on locally sourced products in Denmark would have negative impacts on prices in other European countries, pharmaceutical companies may decide not to adapt their prices as a response to parallel traded competition. We will pay more attention to this issue in Chapter 6.

3.5　The history of parallel trade in Denmark

When Denmark joined the EC in 1973, parallel trade was just about to become a major issue, both for drug companies and for the courts. The first significant verdict on the issue was spoken in 1974 at a trial between Centrafarm and Sterling Drug Inc.

Sterling-Winthrop Drug Ltd. held property rights for product "A" in the UK[46]. The same product was also for sale in the Netherlands with Winthrop B.V. registered as its owner.

44　EFPIA (2006), The Pharmaceutical Industry in Figures, Page 16, Brussels

45　LMI (2006), Facts and Figures 2006: Medicines and Healthcare, P. 88

46　ECJ Court Judgement 15/74, Centrafarm et al. vs. Stanley Drug Inc., European Court of Justice, 1974

Sterling-Winthrop Drug Ltd. and Winthrop B.V. belong to the same holding firm. Using the British brand name, Centrafarm started importing the drug into the Netherlands. Sterling-Winthrop Drug Ltd. brought procedures against Centrafarm for breach of patent and trade mark rights. The European Court of Justice denied Sterling's request, paving the way for parallel trade of patented products within the European Community.

The final statement issued by the European Court of Justice can be summarised as follows: Once a property right holder has sold a product (or given consent for the product to be sold/given away) he should no longer be able to prevent a third party from shipping that product to another country within the EC. The court makes no difference between the property right holder himself, or an authorized license holder who has brought the product into circulation for the first time. Moreover, the court ruled that it is irrelevant whether the price difference between member states is the consequence of government interventions or market forces.

Despite the court ruling of the ECJ, it was 1990, before Denmark authorised parallel imports of pharmaceuticals[47]. Denmark was able to prevent parallel imports of pharmaceuticals because the Centrafarm judges had only presented their view on the exhaustion of intellectual *property rights*. Article 29 of the EC treaty, however, allows member sates to restrict imports on the grounds of the *protection of health*. Policy makers in Denmark had, for a long time, defended the view that parallel trading of pharmaceuticals was not safe. In 1991, Paranova started supplying parallel traded pharmaceuticals to hospitals. By the end of 1991, 61 parallel traded import licenses had already been granted by DKMA[48]. However, parallel traders had difficulties in selling their products to wholesalers and pharmacies for another five years. The principal reasons for this difficult start are listed below:

1. Parallel traders could not apply for a simplified marketing authorisation until 1990
2. Wholesalers had no obligation to buy or sell parallel traded products until 1995
3. Pharmacists had no obligation to buy and sell parallel traded drugs until 1993, when the 5 Kroner substitution rule was implemented[49].
4. Neither wholesalers, nor pharmacists had incentives to buy or sell parallel traded pharmaceuticals until 2001, when discounts were permitted.

Indeed it is only after wholesalers were requested to deal with parallel traded products that market shares picked up markedly[50]. Even though national regulations allow parallel traders to supply pharmacies directly, wholesalers have a gate-keeping function in Denmark too. Unlike classical wholesalers, parallel traders are unable to profitably supply small or remote pharmacies. The reason why parallel traders are unable to install a nationwide distribution network, is the much smaller product portfolio and lower revenues. The average consignment of a classical wholesaler is much larger than the consignment of a parallel trader. It may therefore pay off for the classical wholesalers to supply a smaller or middle sized pharmacy but not for the parallel trader. Forcing wholesalers to deal with parallel traded drugs was a necessity to ensure that parallel traders would have access to the Danish drug market.

---

47 Vallgårda S. et al. (2001), Healthcare Systems in Transition : Denmark, Vol. 8, Nr. 7, Page 67

48 Interview with H. Bøgh-Sørensen et al., Orifarm A/S, Odense, 06.06.2004

49 The substitution rule requires pharmacists to dispense the parallel traded version whenever the price difference between parallel traded and locally sourced products exceeds DEK 5

50 Interview with H. Bøgh-Sørensen et al., Orifarm A/S, Odense, 06.06.2004

By the end of the last decade, market shares of parallel traded pharmaceuticals had reached 10%, where they stabilized.

3.6 Parallel trade in Denmark: an empirical view

3.6.1 Trade volumes

Parallel traders had a difficult start in Denmark. First their market entry was retarded by safety regulations. Then wholesalers prevented them from getting their products to the pharmacist and the end consumer. When trade barriers had finally fallen, however, parallel import penetration picked up markedly, hitting 10% in 1997. In 1999 the authorities passed a bill that limited the Danish price to the average price observed in other EU countries. Following the implementation of the bill, the medicine price index experienced a 12% decline between 1999 and 2003. Despite the reduction of the medicines price index, parallel traders have been able to maintain a market share of approximately 10% through the first half of the decade. Sales of locally sourced and parallel traded pharmaceuticals between 2000 and 2004 are summarized in Table 3.2.

Table 3.2 Sales of locally sourced and parallel traded pharmaceuticals in Denmark at pharmacy purchasing prices

	2000	2001	2002	2003	2004 (-Jul)	2004[e] Full Year
Total pharmaceutical sales, million DKK	7 675	8 434	9 505	10 045	6 004	10 721
Market share of parallel imported drugs, in percent	10.3%	10.4%	9.9%	10.5%	10.5%	10.5%
Parallel imported drugs, sales in million DKK	793	874	945	1 050	631	1 126
	CAGR 00–03	CAGR 01–03	CAGR 02–03	CAGR 00–04[e]	CAGR 02–04[e]	CAGR 03–04[e]
Locally sourced drugs	9.4%	9.1%	5.7%	8.7%	8.3%	6.7%
Parallel imported drugs	9.8%	9.6%	11.1%	9.1%	8.8%	7.2%

[e] own estimates based on reported sales Figures for January through July 2004
Source: DLI – Dansk Lægemiddel Information Sales Database[51], 2004

---

51 The DLI database reports monthly sales figures (total sales for parallel traded and locally sourced drugs [branded and generic] at pharmacy purchasing prices for all active substances (ATC5 code) sold in Denmark)

3.6.2 Information on the competitive situation and the revenues of selected products

For our evaluation we have selected 47 products from 17 ATC4 classes that are for sale in Denmark. The sample includes the twenty-five top selling products in Denmark[52] and their direct competitors[53]. In the years 2003 and 2004, fifteen products were facing generic competition and 46 products were exposed to competition from parallel trade. Parallel trade for Losec, which is also included in our sample, stopped in the year 2002 due to generic competition. In 2003, the forty-seven products accounted for 27% of the Danish drug market. Market penetration of parallel imported drugs within our sample was 23.2% in 2003, compared to 10.5% for the total market. Total revenues of all parallel imported products that are included in our sample accounted for approximately 62% of parallel trade. Market penetration of parallel imported products within the remaining market is 5.4%. Table 3.3 provides an overview of revenues generated by locally sourced and parallel traded brands and generics in 2003. Table 3.4 lists all products that are included in our survey. Products are ordered by therapeutic subgroup, ATC-code, non proprietary and brand name. The last two columns show whether a specific product is exposed to parallel traded or generic competition.

Table 3.3 Information on revenues of the 47 products selected for Denmark

No of products	# of prod. w/comp. from PI	# of prod. w/ gen. competition	
47	46	15	
Overview 2003	**TOTAL**	**NN** **(Branded & GEN)**	**PI**
Sales total market (in m DEK)	10 045	8 995	1 050
% of total market	100%	89.5%	10.5%
Sales sample (in m DEK)	2 739	2 084	655
% of sample	100%	76.1%	23.9%
% of relative market	27.3%	23.2%	62.3%

Source: Own calculations based on DLI – Dansk Lægemiddel Information A/S (2004)

---

52 Provided a parallel traded version was available between 2000 and 2003
53 Direct competitors are all drugs with the identical active substance (same ATC5 code)

Table 3.4 Information on the competitive situation of the 47 products selected for Denmark

ATC4 Group	ATC Code	Generic name	Brand name	Exposed to competition from PI[a]	Exposed to generic competition[a]
Proton Pump Inhibitors	A02BC01	Omeprazole	Losec	N	Y
	A02BC03	Lanzoprazole	Lanzo	N	Y
	A02BC03	Lanzoprazole	Lanzo	Y	N
Calcium Channel Blockers	C07AB02	Metoporol	Seloken	Y	Y
	C07AB04	Acebutol	Diasectral	Y	N
	C07AB05	Betaxolol	Kerlon	Y	N
	C07AB07	Bisoporol	Emonocor	Y	N
Beta Blocking Ag.	C08CA01	Amolidipine	Norvasc	Y	Y
	C08CA02	Felodipin	Felodipin	Y	N
	C08CA03	Isradipine	Lomir	Y	N
	C08CA05	Nifedipine	Adalat	Y	N
ACE II Inhibitors	C09CA01	Losartan	Cozaar	Y	N
	C09CA03	Candesartan	Attacand	Y	N
Beta Blocking Ag.	C10AA01	Simvastatin	Zocor	Y	Y
	C10AA02	Lovastatin	Mevacor	Y	Y
	C10AA03	Pravastatin	Pravachol	Y	N
	C10AA05	Atrovastatin	Lipitor	Y	N
Tetracyclines	J01FA09	Clarithromycin	Klacid	Y	N
	J01FA10	Azithromycin	Zythromax	Y	N
Selective Immuno-suppressives	L04AA01	Ciclosporin	Sandimmun	Y	N
	L04AA05	Tacrolimus	Prograf	Y	N
Coxibs	M01AH01	Rofecoxib	Vioxx	Y	N
Bisphosphonats	M05BA01	Etidronic acid	Didronel	Y	N
	M05BA04	Alendronic acid	Fosamax	Y	N
Selective serotonin (5HT1) agonists	N02CC01	Sumatriptan	Imigran	Y	N
	N02CC02	Naratriptan	Naragran	Y	N
	N02CC03	Zolmitriptan	Zomig	Y	N
	N02CC04	Rizatriptan	Maxalt	Y	N
Tetracyclines	N03AX09	Lamotrigine	Lamictal	Y	N
	N03AX11	Topiramate	Toprimax	Y	N
	N03AX14	Levetiracetam	Keppra	Y	N

Table 3.4 *(continued)*

ATC4 Group	ATC Code	Generic name	Brand name	Exposed to competition from PI[a]	Exposed to generic com- petition[a]
Antipsychotics	N05AH02	Clozapine	Leponex	Y	Y
	N05AH03	Olanzapine	Zyprexa	Y	N
	N05AH4	Quetiapin	Seroquel	Y	N
O. antipsychotics	N05AX08	Risperidone	Risperdal	Y	N
Selective sero- tonin reuptake inhibitors (SSRIs)	N06AB03	Fluxetine	Prozac	Y	N
	N06AB04	Citalopram	Cipramil	Y	Y
	N06AB05	Paroxetine	Seroxat	Y	Y
	N06AB06	Sertaline	Zoloft	Y	Y
	N06AB10	Escitalopram	Cipralex	Y	N
O. Anti- depressants	N06AX16	Venlafaxine	Efexor	Y	N
Antcholinester- ases	N06DA02	Donepezil	Aricept	Y	N
Adrenergics and other drugs for obstructive air- way diseases	R03AK03	Fenoterol	Berodual	Y	N
	R03AK05	Salmeterol	Seretide	Y	N
	R03AK07	Formoterol	Symbicort	Y	N
Glucocorticoids	R03BA02	Budesonide	Pulmicort	Y	N
	R03BA05	Fluticasone	Fluxotide	Y	N

[a] Includes products which were exposed to parallel traded competition/generic competition for the full year of 2003

Source: DKMA, price database, accessed 13.02.2006

http://www.laegemiddelstyrelsen.dk/1024/visLSArtikel.asp?artikelID=1431

3.6.3   Pricing and savings from parallel imported products

a)   Description of the data sample and the methodology

For our evaluation, we use pack specific pricing information for each product included in our sample. Pricing information for every item (active substance, dosage, pack size, brand name, manufacturer [branded/generic] and distributor) is available on the internet portal of the Danish Medicine Control Agency[54]. Prices are updated every two weeks and recorded in a rolling database for five years. Sales figures for all products were provided by DLI, a daughter company of the Danish Association of the Pharmaceutical Industry (LIF DK). The

---

54 http://www.laegemiddelstyrelsen.dk/1024/visLSArtikel.asp?artikelID=1431

database reports monthly sales figures (DDD and PPP) for all active ingredients that are marketed in Denmark. For privacy reasons, DLI was unable to provide us with pack specific sales information. However, we were able to use a Database with substance specific sales information. Products are listed according to their ATC5 code and generic name. For each substance we have monthly sales numbers on locally sourced and parallel traded drugs. Locally sourced drugs may include generics in case the product is off-patent.

Table 3.5 shows an extract of the Datasheet that we used to do the calculations. The first line reports total sales of Amphotericin (Fungizone®) at pharmacy purchasing prices in 1999. The second line reports total sales of locally sourced products. No generic was available for Fungizone® in 1999. Locally sourced drugs generated DKK 90 000 between August and December of the year 1999; parallel traded versions (imported by Paranova and Orifarm) achieved a turnover of DKK 210 000 at pharmacy purchasing prices[55].

Table 3.5 Data sample with sales information on locally sourced and parallel traded Fungizone in Denmark

PPP	1999	1999/Aug	1999/Sep	1999/Oct	1999/Nov	1999/Dec
A01AB04 Amphotericin	300	50	90	90	30	30
A01AB04 Amphotericin No parallelimport	90	20	40	10	10	10
A01AB04 Amphotericin. Parallelimport	210	30	50	80	20	20

Source: Own illustration based on DLI database

Because we lacked pack specific sales information, we were unable to calculate the exact savings resulting from parallel trade in Denmark. We are, nevertheless, able to give an accurate estimate on total savings resulting from parallel imports of pharmaceuticals into Denmark. To achieve the best possible results, we have, for each of the forty-seven products, calculated a proxy for the weighted average price of all parallel traded product versions. Each product is generally sold in various specifications (dosage and pack size). Every specification is marketed by the manufacturer himself and an undefined number of parallel traders. Price gaps between locally sourced and parallel traded drugs are calculated by using the lowest priced product for each specification. Table 3.6 illustrates how we calculated the average price advantage of a parallel traded Pulmicort pack in February of the year 2004. Prices are in DKK per DDD.

In the case illustrated in Table 3.6, PharmaCoDane is the cheapest supplier of the Pulmicort 200 mikg/dose inhaler with 100 doses. For that specific product, PharmaCoDane sets a price of DKK 7.8 per DDD compared to the 9.1 charged by Astra Zeneca, the intellectual

---

55 Please note, that the table is for illustration purposes only: Figures have been modified by the author

property right holder and the DKK 8.6 charged by Orifarm and Paranova. PharamCoDane is therefore the cheapest supplier of the Pulmicort 200 mikg/dose inhaler with 100 doses. PharmaCoDane sets a price which is 13.7% below the price of the locally sourced product. Apart from the Pulmicort 200 mikg/dose inhaler with 100 doses parallel imported substitutes were available for four other specifications of the drug. These products were offered at price advantages of 15.3%, 13.4%, 25%, 3% and 1% by the cheapest supplier in each respective case. The average price advantage for all cheapest suppliers was 12.5%, the value that we use for Pulmicort on that day.

Table 3.6 Data sample for the calculation of the average price spread between locally sourced and parallel traded pharmaceuticals in Denmark

Product name	Dosage	Pack Size	Distributor	02.02.2004
Spirocort	200 mikg/dose	100 doses	Astra Zeneca	9.1
Pulmicort	200 mikg/dose	100 doses	PharmaCoDane	7.8
Pulmicort	200 mikg/dose	100 doses	Orifarm	8.6
Pulmicort	200 mikg/dose	100 doses	Paranova	8.6
Price advantage of:	**Dosage**	**Pack Size**		**02.02.2004**
PharmaCoDane	*200 mikg/dose*	*100 doses*		*13.7%*
ORIFARM	*200 mikg/dose*	*100 doses*		*5.5%*
PARANOVA	*200 mikg/dose*	*100 doses*		*5.5%*
Cheapest supplier	**200 mikg/dose**	**100 doses**		**13.7%**
Cheapest supplier	200 mikg/dose	200 doses		15.3%
Cheapest supplier	400 mikg/dose	100 doses		13.4%
Cheapest supplier	400 mikg/dose	200 doses		25%
Cheapest supplier	0.25 mg/ml	10*2 ml		3%
Cheapest supplier	0.5 mg/ml	20*2 ml		1%
AVERAGE ALL PRODUCTS				12.5%

Source: Own Calculations, based on 5-year rolling price statistics from DKMA, downloaded from: http://www.laegemiddelstyrelsen.dk/1024/visLSArtikel.asp?artikelID=864, in June 2005

**b) Average price advantages and savings
from parallel imported products, monitored market**

The following numbers refer to the 46 products listed in Table 3.3. In the time period between January 1st 2002 and July 31st 2004, the average price gap between a locally sourced and a parallel traded drug was 7.8%. Locally sourced drugs generated sales of DKK 5.4 bn, parallel traded drugs generated sales of DKK 1.6 bn. Market shares of parallel traded products were as high as 24.1%, compared to approximately 10% for the entire market. Savings amounted to DKK 135.4m. Price advantages of parallel traded drugs were highest in the year 2001 (12.3%) and lowest in the first three quarters of the year 2004 (5.4%). Possible savings from discount sharing between pharmacies and the NHS remain unaccounted for in our study. Table 3.7 summarises these results and provides further information on pricing, revenues and savings from parallel traded pharmaceuticals in Denmark.

Table 3.7 Sales of and savings from parallel trade in Denmark in million DKK: data sample

	2000	2001	2002	2003	2004 Jan–Jul	02–04
Total drug sales	2042.1	2319.6	2707.9	2739.8	1535.1	6982.8
Sales locally sourced drugs	1619.5	1827.7	2152.5	2084.9	1148.2	5459.7
Sales parallel imported drugs	422.6	491.9	555.4	654.9	386.9	1597.2
Market share of parallel imported drugs	21.8%	23.5%	22.1%	25.5%	25.1%	24.1%
Price advantage parallel imported drugs	6.2%	12.3%	8.8%	8.4%	5.6%	7.8%
Savings parallel imported drugs	27.8	68.9	53.6	59.8	22.0	135.4

Source: Own calculations based on LIF DK

3.6.4 Average price advantages and savings from parallel trade, total market

The following figures refer to the full time period between January 2002 and July 2004. Parallel traded versions of all products which are included in our sample, generated savings of DKK 135m at pharmacy purchasing prices, as seen in the last column of Table 3.7. The pharmacy purchasing price accounts for 62% of the retail price. At pharmacy distribution prices (VAT incl.) parallel trade has therefore generated savings of DKK 218m. Our sample accounted for 62.3% of total turnover generated by parallel traders. Assuming that the observations on price advantages of parallel traded products are representative for the entire market, total savings from parallel trade would have summed up to DKK 360m or DKK 67 per capita. As a percentage of overall drug expenditures, parallel imports would have induced savings of 0.9%. The numbers mentioned above as well as details on price advantages of and savings from parallel trade for the years 2002 through 2004 are listed in Table 3.8[56].

For the case of Norway and Denmark, we have estimated overall savings from parallel trade by processing pricing and sales information of a selection of high revenue drugs and

---

56 Our own calculation based on pack-specific pricing information (DKMA) and sales data (DLI)

Table 3.8 Benefits from pharmaceutical parallel trade in Denmark (total market at retail prices)

	2002	2003	2004 Q1–Q2	2002–2004 Q2
Sales of locally sourced drugs (million DKK)	13 806.3	14 506.6	8 666.3	36 979.2
Sales of parallel imported drugs (million DKK)	1 524.7	1 695.1	1 017.7	4 237.6
Average price advantage of parallel imported drugs	8.8%	8.4%	5.4%	7.8%
Savings from parallel trade (million DKK)	147.1	154.7	57.9	359.7
Savings from PI as a share of total drug expenditures[a]	1.0%	0.9%	0.6%	0.9%
Penetration rate parallel imported drugs (value)	10.0%	10.5%	10.5%	10.3%
Penetration rate parallel imported drugs (volume)	10.8%	11.3%	11.0%	11.1%
Savings/ capita (DKK)	27.37	28.70	10.70	66.8
Savings /capita (EUR)	3.68	3.86	1.43	8.98

[a] Based on total sales of locally sourced drugs plus sales of parallel traded drugs at locally sourced prices
Source: Own calculations based on DKMA price database and Dansk Lægemiddel Information A/S

extrapolating these numbers to the total market. For Denmark we have figures from the Danish Association of Parallel Traders saying that price advantages of *all* parallel imported pharmaceuticals were at 8.0% (our estimate is 8.4%) in 2003. Our extrapolation led to a slight overestimation of price advantages and therefore savings. *Our* moderate overestimation of savings is therefore a consequence of using the price of the cheapest parallel imported product (per formulation) in order to calculate average savings and selecting high revenue drugs as a proxy for the entire market.

3.7 The impact of competition on the pricing behaviour of parallel traders

In the introductory section of this chapter, we argued, that both the substitution and the reimbursement rule, are appropriate tools to promote price competition among parallel traders and generic manufacturers. We also argued that the price gap between the locally sourced and the parallel traded drug should grow, as additional parallel traders and generic competitors enter the market. Furthermore, we outlined that a higher penetration rate of parallel traded goods would have a beneficial impact on price competition among parallel traders. In the last subsection we noticed that price advantages of parallel traded goods accounted for in our survey, decreased substantially in the year 2004. We find that the turnover of the four parallel traded products, which had been most attractively priced, dropped from DKK 94.1 m in 2003 to just about DKK 6 m in the year 2004. The products in question (Adalat, Zocor, Prozac and Seroxat) had become subject to generic competition in 2002 or before. As generic competitors entered, parallel traders responded by gradually lowering their prices. Parallel traders were able to stand up to generic competition until about 2003, when eroding generic prices forced them to pull out of the market.

It may, therefore, be interesting to compare pricing patterns of parallel traded products which are or are not exposed to generic competition. Table 3.9 shows that between 2002 and 2004, the average price difference between the parallel traded and the locally sourced product not exposed to generic competition was 5.3%. The price difference between the parallel traded and the locally sourced drug which is exposed to generic competition, by contrast was 17.7%. Parallel traded products subject to generic competition generated 46.4% of all savings while accounting for 18.2% of sales only. This is an indicator that the additional presence of generic competition induces parallel traders to offer more competitive prices.

Table 3.9 Savings from parallel traded goods which are or are not exposed to generic competition

	2002	2003	Jan–Jul 2004	01.02– 07.04
With generic competition				
Sales of locally sourced drugs (million DKK)	462.2	496.5	363.5	1 322.2
Sales of parallel traded drugs (million DKK)	150.1	105.1	36.0	291.3
Relative price advantage of parallel traded drugs	14.7%	24.2%	8.8%	17.7%
Savings parallel imported drugs (million DKK)	25.8	33.6	3.5	62.8
Penetration rate parallel imported drugs	27.6%	21.8%	9.8%	21.1%
Sales as a percentage of all parallel traded drugs	27.0%	16.1%	9.3%	18.2%
Savings as a percentage of all parallel traded drugs	48.1%	56.1%	15.8%	46.4%
Without generic competition				
Sales of locally sourced drugs (million DKK)	1 690.2	1 588.4	784.7	4 063.4
Sales of parallel traded drugs (million DKK)	405.3	549.8	350.8	1 305.9
Relative price advantage of parallel traded drugs	6.4%	4.6%	5.0%	5.3%
Savings parallel imported drugs (million DKK)	27.8	26.3	18.5	72.6
Penetration rate parallel imported drugs	20.4%	26.6%	32.0%	25.3%
Sales as a percentage of all parallel traded drugs	73.0%	83.9%	90.7%	81.8%
Savings as a percentage of all parallel traded drugs	51.9%	43.9%	84.2%	53.6%

Source: Own calculations based on DKMA price database and Dansk Lægemiddel Information A/S

If the presence of generics has an influence on the price gap between locally sourced and parallel traded pharmaceuticals, the number of parallel traders may have such an influence too. To verify if an increased number of parallel traders leads to lower drug prices, we have processed pricing information on 47 products. We find evidence that a higher number of parallel traders per original brand, leads to higher price differences between the parallel traded and the locally sourced product. Price differences between the parallel traded and the locally sourced product are highest, when the brand is challenged by generic competition. In the year 2003, parallel imported products where priced 3.3% below the locally sourced drug when being marketed by one parallel trader only. Parallel traded products which were marketed by two traders were priced 4.6% below the locally sourced drug. If the number of parallel traders is three or larger, the average price difference between locally sourced and parallel traded drugs increases to 6.8%.

Table 3.10 Average price advantage of parallel traded goods depending on competition

	1999	2000	2001	2002	2003	2004
One parallel trader	3.3%	3.0%	3.4%	3.0%	3.3%	2.3%
Two parallel traders	2.8%	3.9%	4.6%	3.8%	4.6%	3.8%
Three parallel traders or more	3.7%	6.4%	7.1%	5.3%	6.8%	7.9%
Generic competition	8.8%	13.4%	16.2%	11.6%	31.9%	22.0%

Source: Own calculations based on DKMA, 2004

The figures presented in Table 3.10 suggest that price differences between locally sourced and parallel traded drugs increase with the number of parallel traders and are highest if the brand is challenged by generic competition. In order to verify if these differences between price advantages of parallel traded products are statistically significant we use t-tests of the hypothesis that price advantages are the same.
    We test the hypothesis:

$H_0 : \mu_A - \mu_B = 0$

against the alternative

$H_0 : \mu_A - \mu_B > 0$

at a *minimal* significance level of $\alpha = 0.05$
with A and B representing the number of parallel traders and μ representing the average price gap between locally sourced and parallel traded drugs.

a) Price advantages of products marketed by one parallel trader compared to price advantages of products marketed by two

In the year 2003, the relative price advantage of a parallel traded pharmaceutical marketed by one parallel trader (μ_1) was 3.3% ($\sigma_1 = 0.04972$). The relative price advantage of a pharmaceutical marketed by two parallel traders (μ_2) was 4.6% ($\sigma_2 = 0.06368$). The number of observations is 92 for products which are marketed by one parallel trader and 114 for products which are marketed two parallel traders. These figures are summarized in Table 3.11.

Table 3.11 Group statistics: Price advantages of products marketed by one parallel trader compared to price advantages of products marketed by two (Denmark, 2003)

N° of parallel traders	N° of observations	Unweighted average (μ)	Standard deviation (σ)
1	92	0.0332	0.0497
2	114	0.0455	0.0637

A Levence's test for the equality of variances (F = 1.96, p-value = 0.166) confirms the assumption on the equality of variances. We have therefore run a t-test, assuming *equal variances,* of the hypothesis sketched above. We find that H_0 cannot be rejected at a 5% level as the critical value for $t_{204;0.05} = 1.66$ is larger than the test statistic T = 1.536. It is, nevertheless, possible to reject H_0 at a 10% significance level. We find some evidence that the price advantage of a parallel traded product is higher if the product is marketed by two parallel traders rather than just by one. The results from the test for equality of means as described above are summarised in Table 3.12.

Table 3.12 Independent sample test: Price advantages of products marketed by one parallel trader compared to price advantages of products marketed by two (Denmark, 2003)

	T	df	Sig (1-tailed)	Mean Difference
Equal variances assumed	1.536	204	0.0664	0.01238

b) Price advantages of products marketed by two parallel traders compared to price advantages of products marketed by three and more

In the year 2003, the relative price advantage of a parallel traded pharmaceutical marketed by two parallel traders (μ_2) was 4.6% ($\sigma_2 = 0.06368$). The relative price advantage of a pharmaceutical marketed by three parallel traders or more ($\mu_{\geq 3}$) was 6.8% ($\sigma_{\geq 3} = 0.07668$). The number of observations is 114 for products which are marketed by two parallel traders and 126 for products which are marketed three parallel traders or more. These figures are summarized in Table 3.13.

Table 3.13 Group statistics: Price advantages of products marketed by two parallel traders compared to price advantages of products marketed by three or more (Denmark, 2003)

N° of parallel traders	N° of observations	Unweighted average (μ)	Standard deviation (σ)
2	114	0.046	0.06368
3 and more	126	0.068	0.07668

The Levence's test (F = 4.150, p-value = 0.042) rejects the hypothesis on the equality of variances. We have therefore run a t-test, assuming *unequal variances,* of the hypothesis sketched above. We find that H_0 can be rejected at a 1% level as the critical value for $t_{236;0.01} = 2.35$ is smaller than the test statistic T = 2.428. At a 1% significance level, the price difference between the locally sourced and the parallel traded product can be considered to be larger if the number of parallel traders is three or more rather than just two. The minimal significance level, at which H_0 could be rejected is 0.8%. The test for equality of means is described in Table 3.14.

Table 3.14 Independent sample test: Price advantages of products marketed by two parallel traders compared to price advantages of products marketed by three or more (Denmark, 2003)

	T	df	Sig (1-tailed)	Mean Difference
Equal variances assumed	2.428	236	0.008	0.01238

c) **Price advantages of products marketed by parallel traders only compared to price advantages of parallel traded drugs which are exposed to generic competition too**

In the year 2003, the relative price advantage of a parallel traded pharmaceutical which was not exposed to generic competition ($\mu_{PI\ only}$) was 5.0% ($\sigma_{PI\ only} = 0.06991$). The relative price advantage of a pharmaceutical which was exposed to generic competition ($\mu_{PI\ and\ Gx}$) was 31.9% ($\sigma_{PI\ and\ Gx} = 0.2783$). The number of observations is 332 for products which are marketed by parallel traders only and 73 for products which are marketed by parallel traders and generic manufacturers. These figures are summarized in Table 3.15.

Table 3.15 Group statistics: Price advantages of products marketed by parallel traders only compared to price advantages of parallel traded drugs which are exposed to generic competition too (Denmark, 2003)

N° of parallel traders	N° of observations	Unweighted average (μ)	Standard deviation (σ)
PI only	332	0.050462	0.06991
PI and generics	73	0.318626	0.278287

The Levence's test (F = 543, p-value = 0.0001) rejects the hypothesis on the equality of variances. We have therefore run a t-test, assuming *unequal variances,* of the hypothesis sketched above. We find that H_0 can be rejected at a 1% level as the critical value for $t_{73;0.01} = 2.4$ is smaller than the test statistic T = 8.18. At a 1% significance level, the price difference between the locally sourced and the parallel traded product can be considered to be larger if the branded drug is exposed to generic competition compared to the case where it is not. The test for equality of means is described in Table 3.16.

Table 3.16 Independent sample test: Price advantages of products which are marketed by parallel traders only compared to price advantages of parallel traded drugs which are exposed to generic competition too (Denmark, 2003)

	T	df	Sig (1-tailed)	Mean Difference
Equal variances assumed	8.18	73	0.0000	0.268164

3.8   The impact of generic and parallel traded competition on the pricing behaviour of drug manufacturers

In 2002, the York Health Economics Consortium published a report on parallel trade in Europe. York estimated direct savings from parallel trade in the year 2001 at 120 m DKK[57]. The accuracy of this figure, which is inline with our findings, has later been confirmed by IMS Health[58]. Moreover, the research group led by West and Mahon, found statistical evidence of competition from parallel imports, forcing pharmaceutical manufacturers to lower the prices of the products concerned[59].

West and Mahon reflect that price cuts imposed by the government could be one possible explanation why prices of locally sourced products, which are exposed to parallel trade, eased back more strongly than prices of locally sourced products not exposed to parallel trade. Prior to the year 2000, pharmaceutical companies in Denmark enjoyed free pricing. In 2000 and 2001, the ex-factory price of a reimbursed pharmaceutical could not exceed the average European price. The implementation of the new pricing rule led to substantial price cuts on products that had initially been more expensive than the European price. Moreover, legislation allowed pharmaceutical companies to increase prices of pharmaceuticals that

57 WestP. et al (2003) Benefits to Payers and Patients From Parallel Trade (2002), The York Health Economics Consortium

58 Haigh, J. (2003) Parallel Trade in Europe – Assessing the Reality of Payer and Patient Savings: A Review of the York Health Economics Consortium Report, IMS-Consulting, London, http://www.imshealth.com/ims/portal/front/articleC/0,2777,6599_41382706_43286344,00.html, accessed on 18.02.2006

59 West P. et al (2003) Benefits to Payers and Patients From Parallel Trade (2002), The York Health Economics Consortium

had initially been cheaper than the European price. West and Mahon explain that pharmaceuticals, which are subject to parallel trade, are more likely to be priced above rather than at or below the European price. They conclude that the implementation of the new pricing rule could be a reason why prices of locally sourced pharmaceuticals, exposed to parallel trade, eased back more strongly than prices of locally sourced products not exposed to parallel trade. This, however, does not preclude that competition from parallel trade has affected pricing behaviour of pharmaceutical companies too.

Kanavos and Costa-Font calculate the average price change of locally sourced products which were either exposed to no competition at all, parallel traded competition only or generic competition between 1997 and 2002[60]. They find that prices of originals not facing parallel imports decreased by 13% between 1997 and 2002 while prices of originals facing parallel imports decreased by 7% only[61]. The observation period ends one year after the relaxation of the pricing law in Denmark. Our evaluation of the government pricing database shows[62] that prices of multiple pharmaceuticals were subject to considerable fluctuations between 1999 and 2002. Prices of various products eased back after the implementation of the pricing reform in 1999 and increased again after the relaxation of the pricing law in 2001. Because of budgetary interventions, it is often difficult to decide if a price change observed on a drug which is exposed to parallel trade can be attributed to parallel trade alone or if other factors have also been playing a role.

We have gathered monthly pricing information on 436 locally sourced products which were available between January 2002 and September 2004. 253 packs faced no competition during that time period while 99 were facing competition from parallel traded drugs and 84 were subject to generic competition[63]. Our evaluation shows that compared to the average price in 2002, the average price in 2004 was 1.3% lower for branded drugs without competitors, 1.9% lower for branded drugs facing competition from parallel trade and 11.5% lower for products facing generic competition.

In order to assess whether these differences are statistically significant we use t-tests of the hypothesis:

$$H_0 : \mu_A - \mu_B = 0$$

against the alternative

$$H_0 : \mu_A - \mu_B > 0$$

at a minimal significance level of $\alpha = 0.05$

60 Kanavos P. and Costa-Font J (2005), Pharmaceutical parallel trade in Europe: stakeholder and competition effects, Economic Policy October 2005, Page 778

61 The authors do not specify if that difference is statistically significant or not

62 http://www.laegemiddelstyrelsen.dk/1024/visLSArtikel.asp?artikelID=864, accessed August 2004

63 Own observations based on the 5-year rolling price database from DKMA

with A and B quoting whether products are subject to no, parallel traded or generic competition and μ representing the average price change of a locally sourced product over the time period defined below.

a) Price changes of locally sourced products exposed to no competition compared to price changes of products exposed to parallel traded competition only

Between 2002 and 2004, prices of locally sourced products, which were not subject to any competition ($\mu_{NO\ Competition}$), eased back by 1.3% ($\sigma_{NO\ Competition} = 0.00424$). In the same time period prices of locally sourced products which were exposed to parallel trade ($\mu_{PI\ Only}$) eased back by 1.9% ($\sigma_{PI\ Only} = 0.00617$). The number of observations is 253 for products which were not subject to any competition and 99 for products which were exposed to parallel traded competition only. These numbers are summarized in Table 3.17.

Table 3.17 Group statistics: Price changes of locally sourced products exposed to no competition compared to price changes of products exposed to parallel traded competition only (Denmark 2002–2004)

Competitive situation	N° of observations	Unweighted average (μ)	Standard deviation (σ)
No competition	253	0.013	0.00424
PI Only	99	0.019	0.00617

The Levence's test (F = 0.57, p-value = 0.81) confirms the assumption on the equality of variances. We have therefore run a t-test, assuming *equal variances,* of the hypothesis sketched above. We find that H_0 cannot be rejected at a 5% level as the critical value for $t_{350;0.05} = 1.65$ is larger than the test statistic T = 0.777. The minimal significance level, at which H_0 could be rejected, is 22%. Even though H_0 cannot be rejected neither at a 5 or a 10% significance level, it is not possible to exclude that pharmaceutical companies have reduced their prices as a response to parallel traded competition.

Table 3.18 Independent sample test: Price changes of locally sourced products exposed to no competition compared to price changes of products exposed to parallel traded competition only (Denmark, 2002–2004)

	T	Df	Sig (1-tailed)	Mean Difference
Equal variances assumed	0.777	350	0.22	0.0606

b) Price changes of locally sourced products exposed to no competition compared to price changes of products exposed to generic (and parallel traded) competition

Between 2002 and 2004, prices of locally sourced products, which were not subject to any competition ($\mu_{\text{NO Competition}}$), eased back by 1.3% ($\sigma_{\text{NO Competition}} = 0.00424$). In the same time period prices of locally sourced products which were exposed to generic competition (μ_{Generic}) eased back by 11.5% ($\sigma_{\text{Generic}} = 0.01326$). The number of observations is 253 for products which were not subject to any competition and 84 for products which were exposed to generic (and parallel traded) competition. These figures are summarized in Table 3.19.

Table 3.19 Independent sample test: Price changes of locally sourced products exposed to no competition compared to price changes of products exposed to generic (and parallel traded) competition (Denmark, 2002–2004)

Competitive situation	N° of observations	Unweighted average (μ)	Standard deviation (σ)
No competition	253	0.013	0.00424
Generic competition	84	0.115	0.01215

The Levence's test (F = 55.3, p-value = 0.0001) rejects the hypothesis on the equality of variances. We have therefore run a t-test, assuming *unequal variances*, of the hypothesis sketched above. We find that H_0 can be rejected at a 0.5% level, as the critical value for $t_{237;0.005} = 2.617$ is smaller than the test statistic T = 7.313. We conclude that generic competition had a considerable impact on pricing behaviour of pharmaceutical companies.

Table 3.20 Independent sample test: Price changes of locally sourced products exposed to no competition compared to price changes of products exposed to generic (and parallel traded) competition (Denmark, 2002–2004)

	T	Df	Sig (1-tailed)	Mean Difference
Equal variances assumed	7.313	100	0.0001	0.1017

We find solid statistical evidence of competition from generics forcing pharmaceutical manufacturers to lower the prices of the products concerned considerably. We observe a moderate price reduction on locally sourced products which are exposed to parallel trade during the time period between 2002 and 2004.

The reason why, between 2002 and 2004, generic competition triggered stronger price reactions than parallel traded competition is straightforward. When a generic is sold in place of the brand, the manufacturer loses the full difference between the ex-factory price and marginal costs of production. When a parallel traded drug is sold in place of the locally sourced drug, losses correspond to the difference between the ex-factory price in the destination and the origin country of parallel trade. As manufacturers will always price their products above marginal costs of production, economic losses of giving up market shares to a generic manufacturer are higher than the damage of losing market shares to a parallel trader. Incentives to deter generic competition are therefore stronger than incentives to deter parallel imported competition.

Data presented by West & Mahon, Kanavos & Cost Font and our data suggest the following. Between 1997 and 2004 there were periods when prices of locally sourced products decreased more quickly when being exposed to parallel trade. In the same time frame, there were other periods when prices of locally sourced products decreased more quickly when *not* being exposed to parallel trade. Let us therefore briefly look at the specific properties of drug market regulations and market properties, to get a better understanding of a pharmaceutical company's pricing behaviour.

As we have explained earlier, drug pricing in pharmaceutical markets is not free. Instead, governments are now setting maximal prices by reference to the prices they observe in other countries. The Danish price, for instance, serves as a term of reference for pricing authorities in Norway, Italy, Sweden and Switzerland. The maximal reimbursement price in Switzerland corresponds to the average price observed in Denmark, Germany, Sweden and the United Kingdom. The maximal reimbursement price in Sweden corresponds to the average price observed in Denmark, Finland and Norway. Imagine now that in order to deter parallel imports of a given product A, the Danish subsidiary would have to reduce the Danish price by 20%. As a consequence of the price reduction in Denmark, authorities in Berne, Dublin and Stockholm would request price reductions of up to 7% for patients in their countries. Because of international benchmarking, it is, therefore, often prohibitively expensive to reduce the price in a destination country to an extent that makes parallel trade unprofitable. We will pay more attention to this issue in Chapter 6.

However, for political reasons it may nevertheless be appropriate to reduce the price of a product, which is affected by parallel trade, to a level which is higher than the price charged by the parallel trader. This could be necessary if failing to do so would trigger sanctions by the authorities or negative press in the destination country. Bad press could, for instance, have a negative influence on the prescription behaviour of physicians. By granting *moderate* price reductions on pharmaceuticals which are exposed to parallel trade, the pharmaceutical company can avoid a negative backlash on its Danish business. Moreover, if the price reduction granted to Danish patients is small enough, price authorities in other countries may not respond by imposing a price cut on that product. A 2% reduction on the Danish price, for instance, would only trigger a 0.5% reduction of the average price observed by the Swiss, and a 0.7% reduction of the average price observed by the Swedish authorities. Such small modulations are not necessarily enough to induce authorities in Berne and Stockholm to request a price reduction for the product in question.

Kanavos and Costa-Font observe that between 1998 and 2002 in Denmark, the average price of the locally sourced product exposed to no competition, decreased quicker than the average price of the product exposed to parallel traded competition. If parallel traders had unlimited access to supplies, not reducing the Danish price would lead to the situation where parallel importers hold a market share of 100%. However, because subsidiaries in origin countries of parallel trade are limiting the quantities they sell to domestic wholesalers, parallel traders do not have access to unlimited supplies of products. Parallel trade volumes are, therefore, restricted by the availability of supplies in southern Europe. We will provide further details on why and how this works in Chapter 6 of this dissertation paper. Because of the industries' ability to contain parallel trade by limiting supplies, it may even be possible to increase the price of the product which is exposed to parallel traded competition, in order to compensate for the direct losses resulting from parallel trade.

We conclude that pharmaceutical companies in Denmark take an adaptive approach to parallel traded competition. In some cases, they will grant moderate price reductions on pharmaceuticals which are exposed to parallel traded competition. In other cases, they will defend their price, in order to minimise the losses resulting from parallel trade.

3.9   The impact of competition on the pricing behaviour of parallel traders

Danish pharmacists are requested to always dispense the lowest priced product to their patients. We should therefore expect parallel traders to constantly undersell their competitors. To verify if this is really the case in Denmark, we have chosen a sample of 15 top selling drugs that were for sale in the time period between 1999 and 2004. On a product per product base, we compared the prices set by different parallel traders. Table 3.21 shows that in 42.7% of all cases a parallel trader would set the same price as one or several of his direct competitors. By moderately altering the definition of "identical" to a maximal price difference of 0.2%, we find that the prices set by two different parallel traders were identical in 58.6% of all cases. We have seen numerous examples, where a third trader enters the market, offering a lower price during the first couple of weeks, only to move in-line with his competitors after some time. We have also seen various examples where two or even three parallel traders, kept selling the same product at the same price for periods of up to half a year, without altering the price once. This supports our view that the Danish system sets incentives to define a list price which is 5% below the price of the locally sourced drug and to selectively grant discounts as competition emerges.

Table 3.21 Price differences between parallel traded packs of the same product

	The same = maximal price difference of 0.2%	The same = maximal price difference of 0.1%	Prices are the same
Price is the same	2 713	2 499	1 979
Price is different	1 197	2 131	2 551
% prices are the same	58.6%	53.7%	42.7%

Source: Own Calculations based on DKMA price differences among different parallel traded versions of a same pack

3.10 Special focus

The empirical section of this chapter has generated a number of insights that are surprising at first sight and may require further clarification. The following paragraphs provide answers for some of these questions.

3.10.1 The relation between the number of competitors and the average price gap between locally sourced and parallel traded pharmaceuticals

In Section 3.7 we claimed that prices of parallel imported drugs fall with the number of competitors. We defend our view by comparing price advantages of products that are either marketed by one, two or more parallel traders. An evaluation of our database with 47 products shows that only 30% of all parallel imported products are distributed by more than two importers. Another 30% are marketed by one parallel trader only. This suggests that savings from parallel trade could be higher, if additional parallel traders entered the market. Based on the data presented in Section 3.7, critics may claim that the relation between the number of competitors and savings to the consumer is not that clear.

If the number of competitors had no impact on prices, Denmark could also entrust one single parallel trader to supply the Danish market with lower priced products from other EU member countries. The import monopolist would then set his profit maximizing price following the 5% rule[64]. If the price for a locally sourced product was, for instance, DKK 1 000, the profit maximizing monopolist would consequently set a price of DKK 980. It is only the admission of a second parallel trader that could induce him to lower that price.

To understand why, let us take a step back and review how the reimbursement and substitution law affects patients' and pharmacists' behaviour. Patients are reimbursed up to the level of the lowest priced of all interchangeable products. Cost sensitive patients will consequently switch from the incumbent to the new drug, provided that it is cheaper.

The incentives, which are given to Danish patients, are comparable to those given to HMO enrolees in the US. HMO members pay lower co-payments for preferred than for non preferred drugs. By applying different co-payment levels to different products, HMOs can induce their members to always pick the most cost-effective product. It is therefore reasonable to draw comparisons between the pricing behaviour of generic firms in the US and generic firms and parallel traders in Denmark.

In the last decade, a number of US research papers have demonstrated that generic prices fall with the number of competitors. Frank and Salkever[65] find that with each generic entrant, the average price of generics falls by 5.6% to 7.2%. Thus, on moving from the sample mean of about 3 to 6 competitors, there is a reduction in prices of between 17% and 22%. Reiffen and

---

64 Overview of pricing and reimbursement reforms taken by European countries since 1993, EFPIA, 2003
65 Frank R. and Salkever D. (1997), Generic Entry and Pricing of Pharmaceuticals, J. of Econ. & Mgt. Strategy, 1997, Issue 1, Page 75–90

Ward find that generic drug prices fall with the number of competitors, but remain above long-run marginal costs until there are *eight* competitors or more. They find that the ratio of the generic price to the branded price[66] falls from 0.820 with one generic competitor to 0.762 with two, and continues to decline towards 0.533 as the number of competitors rises[67].

Evidence from the US and our observations in Denmark lead us to the conclusion that the number of competitors has an important influence on prices of generic and parallel traded drugs.

3.10.2   What is keeping additional parallel traders out of the market?

Our research on 46 top selling drugs shows that only 30% of all products for which a parallel traded version is available, are supplied by three importers or more. For another 30%, only one parallel traded substitute is available. This raises the question of why parallel traders stay out of markets which are already supplied by one or two of their competitors. Low market entry and transaction costs should enable parallel traders to import products whose expected revenues are low or average.

To start with, it is important to understand that parallel trading is a quick business. Whenever arbitrage opportunities arise, it is a matter of weeks or perhaps months and not years, until parallel traders start importing that product. When looking at the history of our 47 products, we find that a majority were marketed by one or two parallel traders, during the full four year period, without ever being challenged by a third entrant. We also find that in various cases, the entry of a third or fourth competitor induced the incumbent trader(s) to pull out of that respective market. Empirical evidence from the US generic market shows that more generic firms enter, and enter more quickly in markets with greater expected rents[68]. If the number of parallel importers per brand is low, it is because expected rents are not high enough to attract additional parallel traders.

In the year 2004, total revenues of products sold in Denmark amounted to 1.4 bn EUR at pharmacy purchasing prices[69]. The 75 top selling products accounted for 44.8% of total revenues, leaving just about EUR 772 m in sales to the remaining 1 463 medicinal products which are available in Denmark[70]. The average product of the latter group generates annually revenues of just about EUR 527 700.

Let us now calculate expected revenues and profits from importing such a product, assuming that the parallel trader obtains a market share of 20%, or sales of EUR 105 540. Pedersen et al.[71] find that the average parallel trader mark-up of a product sold in Denmark is 22%. The gross margin of bringing a product with sales of EUR 105 540 into Denmark is consequently EUR 19 000. Costs for receiving and maintaining a marketing authorisation

---

66 Pre-patent expiration
67 Reiffen D. and Ward M. (2002), Generic Drug Industry Dynamics, The Federal Trade Commission
68 Reiffen D. and Ward M. (2002), Generic Drug Industry Dynamics, The Federal Trade Commission
69 EFPIA (2006), The Pharmaceutical Industry in Figures 2006 Edition,
70 http://www.talogdata.dk/sw238.asp, calculation based on the number of directly imported products in Denmark
71 Pedersen M. (2006), The economic impact of parallel import of pharmaceuticals

alone are EUR 2 000 p.a. On top of this, the parallel trader will endure expenses for creating a box and setting up the re-packaging facilities so that the new product can be handled and promoted to wholesalers. It is unlikely that a gross margin of EUR 19 100 p.a. is sufficient to cover all expenses involved in importing such a low revenue drug. This example illustrates that for products accounting for about half of the Danish market, there is not even enough revenue potential for one parallel trader. It is therefore no surprise that parallel traders often choose to stay out of markets where their competitors are already active.

For Zyprexa, Denmark's top selling drug, there are only two parallel traded substitutes. Between 2000 and 2002 only one parallel traded version of the product had been available. Zyprexa received market authorisation in 1996 from the European Agency for the Evaluation of Medicinal Products. At first, Danish Zyprexa sales picked up slowly, making it difficult for a parallel trader to import the product profitably. In November 2000, four years after the registration of the product, Orifarm started selling all formulations at an average price gap of 2% compared to the locally sourced drug. In the year 2000, Zyprexa ranked among the ten top selling products with sales of DKK 112 m (EUR 15 m)[72]. In April 2002 the second and – so far – last parallel trader, Paranova, started selling Zyprexa too. Zyprexa was then the fifth most important drug in terms of sales, generating revenues of DKK 190 m (EUR 25 m). For a period of 17 months, Orifarm had been the only parallel trader offering Zyprexa to Danish consumers. During that period, Orifarm held a market share of 20%.

In 2005, Zyprexa generated sales of DKK 229 m (EUR 30.7 m) at pharmacy purchasing prices. Danish wholesaler prices for locally sourced products were 31% higher than average wholesaler prices in Spain, Greece and France. By supplying the whole market at Danish prices, parallel traders could have generated gross profits of EUR 9.5 m. Regardless of the considerable arbitrage potential offered by Zyprexa, there were only two parallel traders, Orifarm and Paranova, selling Zyprexa in April 2007. We conclude that the revenue potential or the availability of Zyprexa in Southern Europe is too small to attract a third parallel trader. Another interpretation could be that market entry and marginal costs to parallel traders are higher than one would suppose.

3.10.3   Is the observation period not too short to reject the hypothesis of price convergence?

In Chapter 3.8 we calculate price changes of locally sourced products which were either subject to no, parallel traded or generic competition, between 2002 and 2004. Prices of locally sourced products which were not facing any competition eased back by 1.3%, prices of locally sourced products which were facing parallel traded competition eased back by 1.9% and prices of locally sourced products which were facing generic competition eased back by 11.5%. At a 0.5% significance level, we reject the hypothesis that price changes of locally sourced products exposed to no and generic competition are comparable. The hypothesis that price changes of locally sourced products facing no and parallel traded competition are comparable, however, can only be rejected at 22% level. This, however, does not prove that

---

72 DLI – Dansk Lægemiddel Information Sales Database, 2004

between 2002 and 2004, pharmaceutical companies have not adapted their prices to take account of parallel traded competition.

Critics may claim that by choosing a longer observation period, one would have been able to obtain significant results. However, when looking at other literature, we find that choosing an observation period of two to five years is common standard. Ganslandt and Maskus for instance[73] calculate – for Sweden – price changes of locally sourced products between 1997 and 1998. At a 5% significance level, they reject the hypothesis that price changes of locally sourced products facing parallel traded competition were identical to price changes of those facing no competition. Kanavos & Costa-Font[74], West and Mahon[75] and Pedersen et al.[76] chose observation periods of three to five years.

Choosing a two to three year time frame is therefore common standard in research on parallel trade of pharmaceuticals. To understand why, let us look at the average life cycle of a pharmaceutical drug. Patent duration of pharmaceuticals is twenty years. Average time from patent registration to product authorisation by the EMEA, is twelve years. Average delay between market approval by EMEA and effective market access in the typical origin country of parallel trade ranges from 327 days in Spain to 435 days in Belgium[77]. Assuming that parallel trade starts on the day that a product receives market access in the origin country, it will only last another 6 to 7 years until patent expiry. In practice, however, it is unlikely that parallel importers can start trading a product the very same day it becomes available in the low price country.

An evaluation of our dataset from Denmark[78] reveals the following about the availability of our 46 products between January 2000 and July 2004:

- For 41 molecules, the locally sourced brand was available for the full time period. In contrast, a parallel traded brand was only available for the full time period for 23 molecules.
- In 18 cases, parallel traded competitors started selling after their locally sourced rival
- 5 parallel traded products stopped trading before product withdrawal of the locally sourced product
- For the five molecules that received marketing authorisation after January 2000, the average time span between market entry of the locally sourced brand and market entry of its first parallel traded competitor was 18 months.
- In thirteen cases, the parallel traded version of a brand which had already been on sale before January 2000 became available after that date. The average parallel traded product in that subgroup was launched during the second quarter of 2002, at a time when the locally sourced product had already been on the Danish market for at least 2.4 years.

The observations show that no drug is exposed to parallel trade eternally. Parallel imports cannot start before a product has been placed on a market where prices are sufficiently low

---

73 M. Ganslandt, K.E. Maskus (2004), J. of Health Economics 23 (2004) 1035–1057, p.1049

74 Kanavos P. and Costa-Font J (2005), Pharmaceutical parallel trade in Europe: stakeholder and competition effects, Economic Policy October 2005, p 778

75 West P. et al. (2002) Benefits to Payers and Patients From Parallel Trade, The York Health Economics Consortium

76 Pedersen K. et al. (2006), The Economic Impact of parallel import of pharmaceuticals, University of Southern Denmark

77 IMS Health (2006), Pricing and market access review 2006, Page 22

78 DKMA

to allow middlemen to profitably engage in parallel trade. From IMS, we derive that this is now generally the case a year and a half after the launch of a product in Denmark[79]. From that moment it takes approximately six years until patent expiry. After patents have expired, parallel traders are generally forced to withdraw their products due to generic competition. Six years shall, therefore, be regarded as the longest possible period over which a product is exposed to parallel traded competition. Our sample on top selling parallel traded drugs shows that average times over which a pharmaceutical drug is challenged by parallel traded competition are substantially lower. This implies that choosing observation periods which are substantially longer than two to five years, reduces the availability of products that can be included in the sample and reduces the likelihood of obtaining significant results.

It is therefore reasonable to use observation periods of two (Maskus and Ganslandt) to five (Kanavos and Costa-Font) years to assess how the presence of parallel traded products affects the pricing behaviour of pharmaceutical companies.

3.11 Conclusions and proposals for future policy reforms

Savings from parallel trade in Denmark account for approximately 1% of total drug expenditures. Price differences between parallel traded and locally sourced drugs grow inline with the number of parallel traders who are selling the same product at the same time. Relative price advantages of parallel traded drugs are highest if the locally sourced brand is at the same time exposed to generic competition.

We derive that price competition among parallel traders is more intense if parallel trade volumes imported into Denmark are close to or above domestic demand. If parallel trade volumes are far below domestic demand, parallel traders can easily sell their products without setting the lowest price.

Because of product shortages in Southern Europe, it has become more difficult for parallel traders to source the quantities that they would be able to sell in Denmark. Product shortages in Southern Europe make parallel imported products in Denmark more expensive. While there is nothing that Denmark can do about product shortages in the origin countries of parallel trade, there are a number of reforms that could help Danish consumers to benefit more from parallel trade.

The provision that allows pharmacies to retain up to 50% of any discounts they receive, sets incentives to all upstream players to compete by selectively offering discounts to the customers rather than by reducing their list price. The practice of setting a list price and selectively granting discounts is called implicit price discrimination. From the consumers' perspective, this is undesirable because they end up paying higher prices than under uniform pricing. Moreover, Danish patients do save – at most – DKK 1 on every DKK 2 that a pharmacist receives as discounts. Denmark should therefore prohibit any granting of discounts. Moreover, wholesaler and pharmacy margins should be decoupled from the ex-factory price.

---

[79] IMS Health (2006), Pricing and Market Access Review 2006

4

Parallel imports of pharmaceutical drugs into Sweden

4.1 Summary

Sweden joined the European Union in 1994 and facilitated parallel imports of pharmaceuticals as from 1996. The introduction of a simplified authorisation procedure in 1996, combined with the possibility to practice generic substitution, which was later replaced by an obligation to dispense the product of the cheapest supplier (2002), triggered an impressive growth of parallel trade. Today, Sweden is one of the most important destination markets of parallel trade with revenues of SEK 2.1 bn (EUR 230 m) at pharmacy purchasing prices. Parallel import penetration reached 9.3% in 2001 and has stabilized since. Average price advantages of 14.9% on parallel traded drugs lead to savings of 1.6% on the total drug bill for the time period between 2002 and the third quarter of 2004. In value terms, parallel imports of pharmaceuticals have generated savings of EUR 5.0 per capita in 2003, which is twelve times more than what parallel trade is generating in Norway.

Overall, Sweden is the European country where competition among parallel traders is strongest and most beneficial to patients. An evaluation of pricing data on 418 parallel imported boxes shows a clear correlation between the number of competing parallel traders and the price gap between the locally sourced and the parallel traded drug. An evaluation of pricing data on 196 branded boxes which were either subject to no competition, parallel traded competition only or generic competition in the time period between 2001 and 2004, provides strong evidence that generic competition induces branded manufacturers to reduce their prices. Moreover, we find some evidence that the presence of parallel traded competition would induce drug companies to reduce prices in Sweden.

4.2 The Swedish healthcare system

4.2.1 Organization

Healthcare in Sweden is funded, organised and coordinated by the government. National authorities ensure that health services run efficiently and according to their fundamental goals. At a regional level, authorities are responsible for delivering healthcare services and have the authority over the hospitals[80].

---

80 Glenngård A. et al. (2005), Health Systems in Transition: Sweden, Vol. 7 No. 4, Page 18

Primary care is delivered through, publicly owned, primary care centres. Most general practitioners in Sweden are, therefore, salaried employees. Private healthcare providers must have an agreement with the county council in order to be reimbursed from public health insurance. Private healthcare providers receive a mix of salaries, capitation and fee for service payments[81].

Hospitals in Sweden are managed and financed by municipalities. They control the number of hospital beds, the amount of personnel and any investments in new technologies that hospitals make. Most hospitals receive global budgets for their inpatient activities. These budgets are based on past performance and modified at the margin to account for new activities, changes in tasks and areas of specific need. Global budgets are an effective cost containment tool. However, they limit a hospitals flexibility to respond to patient's needs and do not reward efficiency[82].

We conclude that the government controls in- and out-patient expenditures through: the limitation of the number and the selection of healthcare professionals in primary care, the gate keeping function of general practitioners, the ownership and control of the hospital market

Drug manufacturers and parallel traders are privately run, *profit maximizing* businesses. The government cannot dictate to drug manufacturers what product is to be developed. Neither can it tell parallel traders what drugs to offer. They have no direct influence on the availability or the prices of parallel traded pharmaceuticals. Instead, the government has to influence the behaviour of those stakeholders who are prescribing, distributing and buying parallel traded pharmaceuticals. Inducing parallel traders to behave in a desired way is, therefore, more difficult than inducing government controlled hospitals to do the same thing. In the next subchapters we will look at how successful the government is in influencing stakeholders' behaviour.

4.2.2   Reimbursement of pharmaceuticals

Pharmaceuticals in Sweden are divided in two categories: over the counter and prescription drugs. Over the counter drugs are not eligible for reimbursement by the national insurance system, prescription drugs are. Expenditure on prescription drugs is subject to different levels of patient co-payment. The calculation of the reimbursement to patients is based on the total cost of products purchased during the last twelve months. The patient has to pay the full cost for prescribed drugs, up to SEK 900, after which level the subsidy gradually increases to 100%. Within a 12-month period, the maximum co-payment for prescribed drugs is SEK 1 800 (EUR 200). In 2004, the average Swede paid 26% of his personal drug bill out of his own pocket[83]. The average patient has therefore strong financial incentives to switch to lower priced products.

---

81   Glenngård A. et al. (2005), Health Systems in Transition: Sweden, Vol. 7 No. 4

82   Glenngård A. et al. (2005), Health Systems in Transition: Sweden, Vol. 7 No. 4

83   EFPIA (2006), The Pharmaceutical Industry in Figures, Page 37

4.2.3 The price setting process for pharmaceuticals

The Medicines Products Agency (MPA) is responsible for the regulation and surveillance of the development, production and distribution of pharmaceuticals. The Pharmaceutical Benefits Board (LFN) is responsible for deciding whether a new pharmaceutical shall be reimbursed and for negotiating an appropriate pharmacy purchasing and distribution price with the manufacturer. Approved pharmacy purchasing prices are binding, meaning that wholesalers must charge the same price to all pharmacies in the Kingdom of Sweden. It is the responsibility of each wholesaler to negotiate, with his suppliers, a procurement price that allows him to operate profitably.

4.2.4 The distribution chain of pharmaceuticals in Sweden

a) Pharmacies

All pharmacies in Sweden are owned and run by the National Corporation of Swedish pharmacies, Apoteket AB. Apoteket AB is a non- profit, state owned company, that reports to the Ministry of Health. The Ministry of Health is responsible for ensuring that healthcare providers act cost-efficiently. It gives directives to Apoteket on how to ensure a cost effective supply of pharmaceuticals throughout the country. Apoteket's profits are to be reimbursed to its sole shareholder, the Ministry of Health.

Pharmacists working for Apoteket are fixed salaried employees. No bonuses are paid to pharmacists who operate more profitably than their colleagues. Instead, pharmacies are rated on how well cost containment measures are implemented. Whenever there is a directive to dispense a lower priced generic or a cheaper parallel traded brand, pharmacists will do so. Rules, quoting that pharmacies should always dispense the cheapest of all substitutable drugs, are easy to implement where the one who's paying the health bill owns the pharmacies. Pharmacists who work on their own account, however, have incentives to buy and sell the products that allow them to maximize profits.

b) Wholesalers

In Sweden two companies hold licenses to supply medical goods to pharmacies, Kronans Droghandel (KD) and Phoenix. KD is owned by a conglomerate of six leading pharmaceutical companies. Both wholesalers hold a market share of approximately 50%.

Official pharmacy purchasing prices for all reimbursed products are binding and granting of discounts is prohibited on all levels along the distribution chain. Ex-factory prices, however, are free, meaning that manufacturers will preferably sell to the wholesaler who is willing to pay the highest price for a specific product. The system ensures that wholesalers keep their business lean and their distribution cost low.

Swedish wholesalers are not allowed to actively promote certain products. Instead, they are requested to supply the products that pharmacies want. When it comes to the distribution of parallel traded products, wholesalers are requested to buy any quantity that the market will absorb.

When setting a price, pharmaceutical companies and parallel traders will pay more attention to patients' and pharmacists', rather than to wholesalers' considerations.

4.3   How does Sweden encourage parallel traded substitution and competition?

4.3.1   Removing technical trade barriers

a)   Tolerance towards different presentation forms and formulations
In order to meet patient needs, identical products may come along in different forms. The formulation of a product may influence its bioavailability or pharmacokinetics. In other cases, however, the formulation may have no significant impact on the way a product works in the body. Coated pills, for instance, are easier to swallow or better in taste than non-coated pills. The coating substance is generally designed to have no impact on the bioavailability of product. When having developed a new formulation, pharmaceutical companies may decide to gradually replace the old formulation with the new one. In such cases, there may be a transition period where the old formulation is still for sale in some countries but no longer in others. In a prominent lawsuit between Hässle Lækemedel (now Astra Zeneca) and Paranova, the Swedish Courts asked the European Court of Justice how to proceed in such situations.

In that specific case, Hässle Lækemedel held the marketing authorisation in Sweden for "Losec enterokapslar" (hereinafter capsules). Paranova and others held parallel import licenses for the capsules too. At the request of Hässle, the marketing authorisation for the capsules ceased to be valid on January 1st, 1999[84]. Hässle had made the request to terminate the marketing authorisation for the capsules, because it intended to sell a new product version called "Losec MUPS enterotabletter" (hereinafter tablets). Hässle continued selling the capsules in a number of other EU member states under the marketing authorisation granted in these member states. Both product versions are therapeutic equivalents meaning that they contain the same dose of the active ingredient which is absorbed by the body at the same rate and to the same extent when taken orally. Nevertheless, on September 1st, 1998 the Swedish Medicines Control Agency (Läkemedelsverket) decided that the parallel import licenses granted to Paranova and others would expire on the same date as the marketing authorisation which Hässle held. The Läkemedelsverket justified its decision by saying that the capsules and the tablets had to be considered as two distinct medicinal products. Parallel import licenses, however, can only be granted and maintained, if the originator of the drug has a valid marketing authorisation in Sweden. Paranova and others appealed against the decision of Läkemedelsverket.

After several appeals, Swedish Authorities brought the case to the ECJ. The European Court of Justice was requested to decide if it was compatible with Articles 28 and 30 of the EC treaty to revoke a parallel import license if the holder of the marketing authorisation of the directly imported product version had revoked his license for reasons which are not connected with the safety of that product. Moreover, the European Court of Justice was requested to suggest what member states should do in cases where the marketing authorisation for the directly imported version had been replaced by a new license for a product with the same active ingredient but a different formulation (e.g. capsules being replaced by tablets)[85].

---

84   ECJ Case 15/01: Paranova Läkemedel AB et al. vs Läkemedelsverket, European Court of Justice, 2001
85   ECJ Case 15/01: Paranova Läkemedel AB et al. vs Läkemedelsverket, European Court of Justice, 2001

On December 21st, 2001, the European Court of Justice ruled that a withdrawal of the marketing authorisation of the directly imported product version, which came about at request of the property right holder, should not automatically entail the termination of the import license for the parallel traded version. However, if there is in fact a risk to the health of humans as a result of the continued existence of the license for the old product, authorities should have the possibility to revoke the parallel import license.

Today, parallel traders in Sweden are requested to describe any difference between the locally sourced and the parallel traded product version in their application. It is the duty of the MPA to decide if these differences are of therapeutic significance or not. The MPA applies the same standards to parallel traded products as to requests for change of the locally sourced product version. Interviews conducted with parallel traders suggest that MPA has now adopted a pragmatic policy. The agency allows parallel traders to import products which are only equivalent, but not identical to the locally sourced version.

b) Tolerance towards pack size deviations
All products, which are subsidised by public health insurance, are published on a reimbursement list. This list sorts products by non-proprietary name, brand name, form, pack size and dosage. Because of different regulatory requirements or changing marketing strategies pack sizes for identical products are often not the same in Sweden and other European countries. In order to facilitate parallel trade, Swedish authorities have set the standard that parallel trade applications shall be granted in case the pack size of the parallel traded drug is different than the pack size of the locally sourced drug. Prices for pharmaceuticals are published on a Swedish Kroner per Daily Defined Dosage base in order to ensure comparability of prices for products with different pack sizes. Trimming of blisters is permitted, though not appreciated.

c) Trademark and patent law issues
The generic substitution law requires pharmacies to always dispense the cheapest of all interchangeable products unless the physician or the patient objects. All products with the same active substance, dosage and bioavailability are considered to be bioequivalent, irrespective of their brand name. It is, therefore, possible for a parallel trader to sell a product whose brand name does not match the brand name of the equivalent locally sourced product.

Before selling a product, parallel traders need to receive approval for the name they intend to use. Parallel traders may choose between the brand name of the locally sourced product, the non-proprietary name and another name (i.e. the foreign brand). Parallel traders are also allowed to use the Swedish brand name if another name is used in the country where the parallel trader has acquired the product. Interviews with parallel traders confirm that the general strategy is to use the Swedish brand name. Indeed, of the 202 products marketed by Paranova on May 7th, 2004, only six carried the generic name[86]. Cross-Pharma, one of the largest importers in Sweden, used the Swedish brand name for over 95% of its products[87]. Swedish legislation leaves it to the parallel trader, whether to over-stick the original box or to create a new one[88].

---

86 http://www.paranova.se Accessed on May 7th, 2004

87 http://www.crosspharma.se, Accessed on May 7th, 2004

88 Interview with Fredrik Persson, May 27th, 2004

The combination of a strict substitution law and a relaxed policy on property rights, allows parallel traders in Sweden free market access.

d) Conclusions
Product related entry hurdles have not been a big issue in Sweden's parallel trade history. The assessment, whether a parallel import license can be granted to a product is solely based on therapeutic equivalence or bioequivalence. A license is granted, whenever both versions produce essentially the same biological availability of the active substance in the body when taken in the same quantity. Trimming of blisters is not appreciated for product safety and traceability reasons. Parallel traders are, nevertheless, allowed to import packs with sizes which are unavailable in Sweden. Drug manufacturers are consequently unable to segment markets by selling smaller or larger packs to consumers in Sweden.

A relaxed view on property rights and a pragmatic approach on patient safety issues allow parallel traders unrestricted access to the Swedish drug market.

4.3.2 Providing financial incentives to patients to buy lower priced products

In Sweden, the calculation of the reimbursement to patients is based on the total cost of products purchased during the last twelve months. No subsidy is granted as long as total costs do not exceed SEK 900. When the total costs exceed that amount, patients are reimbursed 50 percent of the portion exceeding SEK 900 but less than SEK 1 700, 75 percent of the portion exceeding SEK 1 700 but less than SEK 3 300, 90 percent of the portion exceeding SEK 3.300 but less than SEK 4 300 and 100 percent of total cost exceeding SEK 4 300.

Swedish pharmacies are requested to substitute the locally sourced brand with the lowest priced of all interchangeable drugs which are currently available. It is the patient's right to select another product, provided that he pays the full price difference out of his own pocket. It is then irrelevant if a patient has already exceeded his SEK 1 800 co-payment cap.

In Sweden, prices of all products are freely available on the internet and upon request at LFN. Patients are, therefore, able to check for lower priced alternatives and request a cheaper parallel traded or generic product from their pharmacist. Informed and price conscious end consumers are an important condition for price competition among parallel traders. Both conditions are met in Sweden.

4.3.3 Giving directives to pharmacists to dispense lower priced products

If a drug, which is included in the Pharmaceutical Benefits Scheme has been prescribed and there is one or more substitutable product available, pharmacists are requested to dispense the least expensive one[89]. A drug may not be substituted if the prescriber has objected to it

---

89 Bouvy F. (2003) Overview of pricing and reimbursement measures taken since January 1993, Working Document, EFPIA, Brussels

on medical grounds. Interviews with parallel traders and representatives of the pharmaceutical industry suggest that the box is ticked on approximately 5% of all prescriptions[90]. If the prescriber has objected to substitution, patients do not have to pay the surcharge.

A new ordering system introduced in 2003, highlights the lowest priced of all interchangeable drugs which are currently available, whenever the pharmacist enters the brand of the non-proprietary name of a product into the system. With the new ordering system, it is no longer possible for a pharmacist to order any other than the lowest priced drug, by mistake. Moreover, it saves pharmacists time. Pharmacists who intend to order a more expensive product need to un-tick the product which is suggested by the system before selecting the product of their choice.

The new ordering system is therefore a powerful tool for inducing competition and drive prices down.

4.4 Stakeholder behaviour analysis

The extent to which a country can benefit from allowing parallel imports depends on the behaviour of all stakeholders involved in producing, trading, consuming and financing pharmaceuticals. This chapter looks at the principal stakeholders and how they are expected to behave in Sweden's regulatory and market environment.

4.4.1 Patient behaviour

The current reimbursement system sets incentives to buy the cheapest of all interchangeable products. Interchangeable products are pharmaceuticals with the same active substance, dosage and pharmacokinetics. We shall therefore expect Swedes to insist on receiving the cheapest of all parallel traded or generic product versions, thus putting pressure on pharmacists to have these drugs available in their outlet.

4.4.2 Pharmacists' behaviour

Pharmacists are requested to always dispense the cheapest of all interchangeable products. Pharmacies use a centralised purchasing system. All orders can be monitored by the headquarters of Apoteket AB and the Swedish Ministry of Health. Apoteket's mandate is to ensure a cost effective supply of pharmaceuticals throughout the country. The substitution law is a key element of the Ministries' cost containment policy. Managers and pharmacists working for Apoteket are judged by how successful they are in ensuring that Swedes have cost effective access to medicine. We would therefore expect pharmacists to respect the substitution law and always have the lowest priced of all interchangeable products in their store. When filling a prescription, they will always dispense the lowest priced, of all interchangeable products.

---

90 Interview with Fredrik Persson, May 27th, 2004 and Olle Hageberg, October 2004

4.4.3 Wholesalers' behaviour

Commercial freedom of Sweden's wholesalers is highly restricted. They are facing a monopsonist buyer, who has directives to buy from the lowest priced supplier. Pharmacy purchasing and distribution prices of medicinal products are negotiated between manufacturers and LFN. List prices for all pharmaceuticals are made available by the LFN in a pricing database. These prices are binding for wholesalers, meaning that they cannot charge a price other than the one stipulated by LFN. Wholesaler purchasing prices are negotiated between wholesalers and their suppliers. These prices are set in a way which allows wholesalers to cover their fixed capital and marginal distribution costs. Wholesalers are under pressure to always have the lowest priced of all interchangeable products available. The current legal system forces wholesalers to always buy and dispense the lowest priced of all interchangeable drugs and to operate at low margins.

4.4.4 Behaviour of parallel traders

Act (2002:160) on Pharmaceutical Benefits requires pharmacists to dispense the lowest priced of all interchangeable products[91]. Wholesalers have therefore strong incentives to buy from the cheapest provider in order to be able to supply the drugs that pharmacies want. This exerts pressure on parallel traders to compete with prices. Parallel trading companies are run as rational, profit maximising businesses that will always set the profit maximising price, just as any other firm would do. They will only grant price reductions, if competition or government interventions require them to do so.

We expect the average price gap between parallel traded and locally sourced drugs to grow inline with the number of parallel traders. The reason for this is quite simple. In order to be a wholesaler's preferred provider, a parallel trader has to offer his product at the lowest price. If several parallel traders are actively marketing the same product, wholesalers will first buy from the cheapest provider. Once the cheapest provider is out of stocks, wholesalers will order from the next more expensive provider. Once all parallel traders have run out of stocks, wholesalers will order from the licensed importer.

Rational parallel traders are inclined to lower their prices if they are unable to sell their products. Such situations are more likely to occur if cumulated stocks of parallel imported products are close to, at or even above demand. If cumulated stocks are far below domestic demand, a parallel trader can easily sell his products even when charging a higher price than his direct competitors. We recap that the price gap between parallel traded and locally sourced drugs increases with the number of competing parallel traders and the combined market share of all parallel traders.

Due to stronger incentives to switch to lower priced products and the prohibition of discounts, we should expect price competition to be stronger in Sweden than in the two other countries.

---

91 The Swedish Pharmacuetical Benefits Board (2002), Act (2002:160) on Pharmaceutical Benefits, Section 21 http://www.lfn.se/upload/English/ENG_Act_2002-160.pdf

4.4.5 Behaviour of pharmaceutical companies

Swedish sales organizations of multinational companies are requested to set the price that maximizes corporate profits. The chapters on Norway and Denmark have shown that from the perspective of the local sales organization of a multinational corporation, parallel trade is more harmful than from the perspective of the corporation as a whole. For that reason, requests posted by national sales organizations to reduce prices as a response to parallel trade, are often rejected by the global headquarters. Sweden's pharmaceutical market is 85% larger than the Danish market[92]. Swedish prices for top selling pharmaceuticals are 12% above the Norwegian level[93]. Let us use the example of product X from the last two chapters to see how this affects the corporations pricing decision.

- Total expenditures on product X are capped at EUR 95.25 m p.a.
- Physicians prescribe X until the whole budget is utilized
- Product X is priced at EUR 56 in Sweden and EUR 40 in Greece, where all parallel traded boxes are sourced.
- Transaction costs for creating a new box and importing the product into Sweden are EUR 4
- The drug manufacturer can repel parallel traders from the Norwegian market by charging EUR 44 to Swedish wholesalers
- Marginal production costs per unit of X are EUR 25
- If the manufacturer decides to accommodate parallel trade, parallel traders set a price of EUR 50

By inserting Swedish prices and budget restrictions into Functions 2.1 through 2.4, we find that the Swedish marketing authorisation would choke parallel trade by setting a price of EUR 44, whenever market shares of parallel imported products exceed 22%. From the perspective of the corporation as a whole, however, it is unreasonable to do so before parallel imported products have exceeded a market share of 48.8%. Out of the 26 products which are included in our survey, parallel import penetration was higher than 48.8% in five cases in 2004. However, because price cuts on locally sourced products in Sweden would have negative impacts on prices in other European countries, pharmaceutical companies may, nevertheless, decide not to adapt their prices as a response to parallel traded competition. We will pay more attention to this issue in Chapter 6.

4.5 Parallel trade in Sweden: an empirical view

4.5.1 Trade volumes

Parallel trading of pharmaceuticals into Sweden became possible in 1996; two years after the country had joined the EU. Just as in many other countries, parallel traders started by supplying hospitals, which were eager to buy lower priced products. Pharmacists, however,

---

92 EFPIA (2006), The Pharmaceutical Industry in Figures, Page 16
93 Legemiddelindustriforeningen, LMI (2006), Facts and Figures 2006, Page 88

were reluctant towards buying parallel traded pharmaceuticals, not knowing how patients would react to foreign products. Furthermore, pharmacists had questions regarding the legality of dispensing parallel traded products to the patient. It required a statement by the head of Apoteket AB, that dispensing parallel imported pharmaceuticals was not only legal, but also desirable, before parallel traders received market access in Sweden[94]. Once pharmacies started selling parallel traded products, market shares picked up markedly from 1.9% in 1997 to 9.3% in 2001. In the first half of the current decade, market shares of parallel traded drugs have stabilised at 10% approximately. Sales of parallel traded pharmaceuticals were more than nine times higher in 2004 (SEK 2.5 bn) than in 1997 (269 m). These figures are summarized in Table 4.1.

Table 4.1 Sales of locally sourced and parallel traded pharmaceuticals in Sweden at pharmacy purchasing prices 1997–2004

	1997	2000	2001	2002	2003	2004
Total pharmaceutical sales, m SEK	14 263	20 259	21 647	23 252	23 689	24 234
Parallel imported drugs, m SEK	269	1 749	2 011	2 085	2 099	2 525
Market share of parallel imported drugs, in %	1.9%	8.6%	9.3%	9.0%	8.9%	10.4%
	CAGR 97–04	CAGR 00–04	CAGR 01–04	CAGR 02–04	CAGR 03–04	
Total pharmaceutical sales	7.9%	4.6%	3.8%	2.1%	2.3%	
Sales of parallel imported drugs	37.7%	9.6%	7.9%	10.0%	20.3%	

Source: LIF (2005); FAKTA 2005, Pharmaceutical Market and Health Care

4.5.2   Description of the dataset[95]

For our evaluation we have selected 26 products from 15 ATC4 classes that are for sale in Sweden. In 2003, five products were exposed to generic competition and 25 to parallel traded competition. The 26 products accounted for 20.6% of the Swedish drug market. Market penetration of parallel imported drugs within our sample was 20.7%, compared to 8.9% for the total market. Total revenues of all parallel imported products included in our sample

---

94 Interview with Fredrik Persson, May 27th, 2004

95 Monthly Sales (Revenue in SEK and Volume in DDD) for 26 top selling products (sorted by active substance [ATC5 code], supplier, pack size and dosage) for the time period from January 2001 through October 2004 provided by Läkemedelstatistik, Stockholm

Table 4.2 Information on sales and the competitive situation of the 26 products selected for Sweden

ATC4 Group	ATC code	Generic name	Brand name	Subject to competition from PI [a]	Subject to generic [b] competition
Proton Pump Inhibitors	A02BC01	Omeprazole	Losec	Y	Y
	A02BC03	Lansoprazole	Lanzo	Y	N
	A02BC05	Esomeprazole	Nexium	Y	N
Ca. Channel Blockers	C07AB02	Metoporpol	Seloken	Y	Y
Beta Blocking Ag.	C08CA01	Amlodipin	Norvasc	Y	N
ACE II Inhibitors	C09CA01	Losartan	Cozaar	Y	N
	C09CA03	Candesartan	Attacand	Y	N
Cholesterol Lowering Agents	C10AA01	Simvastatin	Zocor	Y	Y
	C10AA03	Pravastatine	Pravachol	Y	N
	C10AA05	Atrovastatin	Lipitor	Y	N
Tetracicline	J01FA09	Klaritromycin	Klazid	Y	N
	N03AX	Azitromycin	Zytromax	Y	N
Selective Immuno-suppressives	L04AA01	Cyclosporin	Sandimmun	Y	N
	L04AA05	Takrolimus	Prograf	Y	N
	L04AA06	Mykofenol A.	Cellcept	Y	Y
Coxibs	M01AH01	Rofecoxib	Vioxx	Y	N
Byphosphonats	M05BA04	Alendronat	Fosamax	N	N
Antipsychotics	N05AH03	Olanzapin	Zyprexa	Y	N
	N05AX08	Risperdone	Risperdal	Y	N
Selective serotonin re-uptake inhibitors (SSRIs)	N06AB04	Citalopram	Cipramil	Y	Y
	N06AB06	Sertralin	Zoloft	Y	N
O. Antidepressants	N06AX16	Venlafaxin	Effexor	Y	N
Anticholinesterases	N06DA02	Donepezil	Aricept	Y	N
Adrenergics and other drugs for obstructive airway diseases	R03AK06	Salmeterol	Seretide	Y	N
	R03AK07	Formoterol	Symbicort	Y	N
Glucocorticoids	R03BA02	Budesonide	Pulmicort	Y	N
Overview 2003	**TOTAL**	**Locally sourced**	**PI**	**Gx**	
Sales total market (in m SEK)	23 689	18 723	2 099	2 867	
% of total market	100%	79%	8.9%	12.1%	
Sales sample (in m SEK)	4 869	3 379	1 009	281	
% of Sample	100%	73.5%	20.7%	5.8%	
% of relative market	20.6%	19.1%	48.1%	9.8%	

[a] Includes products which were exposed to parallel traded competition during the full year of 2003
[b] Includes products which were exposed to generic competition during the full year of 2003
Source: Own calculations based on LIF/LS, 2005

accounted for approximately 48% of parallel trade. Market penetration of parallel imported products within the remaining market is 5.4%. Data is grouped by active substance, dosage, pack size and supplier. We can, therefore, calculate direct savings from parallel traded product A, with dosage B and pack size C supplied by parallel trader D in month E of year F. Table 4.2 lists all products that are included in our survey. Products are grouped by therapeutic subgroup, ATC-code, non proprietary and brand name. The last two columns show whether a specific product is exposed to parallel traded or generic competition. The lower third of Table 4.2 provides an overview of revenues generated by locally sourced and parallel traded brands and generics in 2003.

4.5.3   Average price advantages

The following figures refer to the 26 products listed in Table 4.2 of this chapter. In the time period between January 1st 2002 and September 30th 2004, the average price gap between a locally sourced and a parallel traded drug was 14.9%. Locally sourced and branded drugs generated sales of SEK 10.2 bn, parallel traded drugs generated sales of SEK 3.2 bn. Market share of parallel traded products was as high as 22.8%, compared to approximately 10% for the entire market. Savings from parallel imports amounted to SEK 530.2 m. Price advantages of parallel traded drugs were highest in the year 2002 (15.7%) and lowest in 2003 (13.8%).

Table 4.3 Price advantages of and savings from parallel traded goods in Sweden (sample)

	2002	2003	01–09.04	2002–2004
Sales locally sourced drugs (million SEK)	4 271.6	3 578.7	2 367.7	10 218.2
Sales parallel imported drugs (million SEK)	971.5	1 009.9	1 043.4	3 024.7
Savings parallel imported drugs (million SEK)	181.1	162.1	187.0	530.2
Sales PT at prices of locally sourced drugs (million SEK)	1 152.6	1 172.0	1 230.4	3 555.0
Price advantages PI	15.7%	13.8%	15.2%	14.9%
Value share PI	18.2%	20.7%	28.4%	22.8%
Volume share PI[a]	20.6%	21.2%	24.9%	25.8%

[a] All products including generics
Source: Own calculations based on LIF/LS 2004

Data confirms that a better market and regulatory environment in Sweden leads to a more intense competition among parallel traders. There are several reasons why competition among parallel traders is more intense in Sweden than in the two other Scandinavian countries.

First, Sweden has a monopsonist pharmacy chain that reports to the same agency which is paying for the drug bill. Second, Sweden does not allow the granting of discounts which can then be diverted into the wallets of wholesalers and pharmacists. Third, the Swedish drug market is twice as large as the Danish or the Norwegian market. This allows a higher number of parallel traders to operate profitably. More parallel traders translate into more competition and lower prices. Fourth, pharmacists are requested to dispense the lowest priced of all interchangeable products and fifth, patients are reimbursed up to the level of the lowest priced of all interchangeable products.

4.5.4 Estimates on total savings from parallel trade

The following figures refer to the full time period between January 2003 and December 2003. The parallel traded versions of all products which are included in our sample, generated savings of SEK 162 m at pharmacy purchasing prices, as seen in the second column of Table 4.3. The pharmacy purchasing price accounts for 83% of the retail price. Our sample accounted for 48% of total sales of parallel traded products in Sweden. Assuming that the observations on price advantages of parallel traded products are representative for the entire market, total savings from parallel trade would have summed up to SEK 406 m or SEK 45 per capita. As a percentage of overall drug expenditures, parallel imports would have induced savings of 1.4%. According to the Swedish Association of Parallel Traders, parallel imported pharmaceuticals were priced 13% below locally sourced drugs in 2003 (our estimate is 13.8%). The association uses pricing and revenue information for every single parallel traded box in Sweden. This suggests that average price advantages of parallel traded products are higher for pharmaceuticals with higher turnovers. These products are more contested. Moreover, parallel traders can, by making use of economies of scale, offer lower prices on high revenue drugs.

In Table 4.3 we see that the average parallel traded product included in our survey was priced 15.2% below the locally sourced drug in the first three quarters of the year 2004. Throughout the full year, sales of parallel traded products amounted to 3.0 bn SEK. Assuming that price advantages of parallel traded products included in our sample are representative for the entire market, total savings for the full year would have amounted to SEK 545.3 m. The numbers mentioned above as well as details on price advantages of and savings from parallel trade for the years 2002 through 2004 are listed in Table 4.4[96].

4.5.5 The impact of competition on the pricing behaviour of individual traders

Chapter 3 has shown that in Denmark, there is a relation between the price advantage of parallel traded products and the number of parallel traders who are selling the same product at the same time. In order to verify if such a relation can be observed in Sweden too, we have

---

96 Our own calculation based on pack-specific pricing information and sales data provided by LIF/LS

Table 4.4 Benefits from pharmaceutical parallel trade in Sweden (total market at retail prices in m SEK)

	2002	2003	2004	2002–2004
Sales locally sourced products	25 502	26 012	26 155	77 669
Sales parallel imported products	2 512	2 529	3 042	8 083
Savings parallel imported products	468.4	406.0	545.3	1 419
Savings parallel imported products per head (SEK)	52.48	45.33	60.52	158.3
Savings parallel imported products per head (EUR)	5.73	4.96	6.63	17.3
Relative price advantage parallel imported products	15.7%	13.8%	15.2%	14.9%
Savings from PI as a share of total drug expenditures	1.7%	1.4%	1.7%	1.6%
Market share of parallel imported drugs (value terms)	9.0%	8.9%	10.4%	9.5%
Market share of parallel imported drugs (volume terms)	10.5%	10.1%	12.1%	10.9%

Source: Own calculations based on LIF 2004

processed pricing information on 26 products. We find that in the years 2001 and 2002 there was no clear relation between the number of parallel traders offering a product and the price difference between the locally sourced and the parallel traded product version. In 2002, the non-weighted price difference between the locally sourced and the parallel traded version was 9.9% for products which were marketed by one single parallel trader, compared to 8.6% for products marketed by four parallel traders.

In 2004, the average price gap between the locally sourced and the parallel traded product was 5.3% for pharmaceuticals being marketed by one parallel trader, compared to 7.6% for products being marketed by two, 11.9% for products being marketed by three and 19.1% for products being marketed by four traders or more. We find that the price gap between the locally sourced and the parallel traded product is higher than in Denmark at all competitive levels, where the price gap between the locally sourced and the parallel traded product was 2.3% for products marketed by one, 3.8% for products marketed by two and 7.9% for products marketed by three parallel traders or more. These figures suggest that parallel traded products in Sweden are priced more attractively than in Denmark under comparable competitive situations. Moreover, we find that the average number of parallel imported versions per product is higher in Sweden than in Denmark. Table 4.5 presents an overview of the price advantages of parallel traded products given specific competitive situations.

In order to verify if the increased price advantages for parallel traded products, which are subject to more intense competition (i.e. further parallel traders or a generic entrant) are statistically significant, we use t-tests of the hypothesis that price advantages are the same.

Table 4.5 Average price advantage of parallel traded goods in Sweden, depending on competition

	2001	2002	2003	2004	2003/04
One parallel trader	9.7%	9.9%	7.8%	5.3%	6.8%
Two parallel traders	8.3%	10.7%	8.2%	7.3%	7.6%
Three parallel traders	13.0%	10.8%	10.7%	13.0%	11.9%
Four parallel traders or more	12.0%	8.6%	17.3%	21.5%	19.1%
Generic competition	17.5%	20.6%	10.9%	13.2%	11.6%

Source: Own calculations based on Läkemedelstatistik:

We test the hypothesis:

$H_0 : \mu_A - \mu_B = 0$

against the alternative

$H_0 : \mu_A - \mu_B > 0$

at a *minimal* significance level of $\alpha = 0.05$
with A and B representing the number of parallel traders and μ representing the average price gap between locally sourced and parallel traded drugs.

a) **Price advantages of products marketed by one parallel trader
compared to price advantages of products marketed by two**
In the two years 2003 and 2004, the relative price advantage of a parallel traded pharmaceutical marketed by one parallel trader (μ_1) was 6.9% ($\sigma_1 = 0.04874$). The relative price advantage of a drug marketed by two parallel traders (μ_2) was 7.6% ($\sigma_2 = 0.05232$). The number of observations is 287 for products which were marketed by one parallel trader and 292 for products which were marketed by two. These figures are summarized in Table 4.6.

Table 4.6 Group statistics: Price advantages of products marketed by one parallel trader compared to price advantages of products marketed by two (Sweden, 2003/2004)

N° of parallel traders	N° of observations	Unweighted average (μ)	Standard deviation (σ)
1	287	0.0685	0.04874
2	292	0.0764	0.05232

A Levence's test for the equality of variances (F = 2.519, p-value = 0.133) confirms the assumption on the equality of variances. We have, therefore, run a t-test, assuming *equal variances*, of the hypothesis sketched above. We find that H_0 can be rejected at a 5% level as the critical value for $t_{577;0.5} = 1.65$ is smaller than the test statistic T = 1.872. The minimal significance level, at which H_0 could be rejected, is 3.2%. Our model confirms that the market entry of a second parallel trader leads to lower prices for the consumer.

Table 4.7 Independent sample test: Price advantages of products marketed by one parallel trader compared to price advantages of products marketed by two (Sweden, 2003/2004)

	T	df	Sig (1-tailed)	Mean Difference
Equal variances assumed	1.87	577	0.032	0.0078

b) Price advantages of products marketed by two parallel traders compared to price advantages of products marketed by three

In the two years 2003 and 2004, the relative price advantage of a parallel traded pharmaceutical marketed by two parallel traders (μ_2) was 7.6% ($\sigma_2 = 0.05232$). The relative price advantage of a pharmaceutical marketed by three parallel traders (μ_3) was 11.9% ($\sigma_3 = 0.07389$). The number of observations is 292 for products which are marketed by two parallel traders and 559 for products which are marketed three parallel traders. These figures are summarized in Table 4.8.

The Levence's test (F = 21.3, p-value = 0.0001) rejects the hypothesis on the equality of variances. We have therefore run a t-test, assuming *unequal variances,* of the hypothesis sketched above. We find that H_0 can be rejected at a 1% level as the critical value for $t_{774;0.01} = 2.3$ is smaller than the test statistic T = 8.860. Our model confirms that the market entry of a third parallel trader leads to lower prices for the consumer.

Table 4.8 Group statistics: Price advantages of products marketed by two parallel traders compared to price advantages of products marketed by three (Sweden, 2003/2004)

N° of parallel traders	N° of observations	Unweighted average (μ)	Standard deviation (σ)
2	292	0.0764	0.05232
3	559	0.1194	0.07389

Table 4.9 Independent sample test: Price advantages of products marketed by two parallel traders compared to price advantages of products marketed by three (Sweden, 2003/2004)

	T	Df	Sig (2-tailed)	Mean Difference
Equal variances assumed	8.860	774	0.001	0.04304

c) Price advantages of products marketed by three parallel traders compared to price advantages of products marketed by four and more

In the two years 2003 and 2004, the relative price advantage of a parallel traded pharmaceutical marketed by three parallel traders (μ_3) was 11.9% ($\sigma_3 = 0.07389$). The relative price advantage of a pharmaceutical marketed by four parallel traders or more ($\mu_{\geq4}$) was 19.1% ($\sigma_{24} = 0.0995$). The number of observations is 559 for products which are marketed by three parallel traders and 1 683 for products which are marketed four parallel traders or more. These numbers are summarized in Table 4.10.

Table 4.10 Group statistics: Price advantages of products marketed by three parallel traders compared to price advantages of products marketed by four and more (Sweden, 2003/2004)

N° of parallel traders	N° of observations	Unweighted average (μ)	Standard deviation (σ)
3	559	0.119	0.07389
4 and more	1 683	0.191	0.09947

The Levence's test (F = 84.7, p-value = 0.0001) rejects the hypothesis on the equality of variances. We have, therefore, run a t-test, assuming *unequal variances,* of the hypothesis sketched above. We find that H_0 can be rejected at a 1% level as the critical value for $t_{1278;0.01} = 2.33$ is smaller than the test statistic T = 18.2. Our model confirms that the market entry of a fourth parallel trader leads to lower prices for the consumer.

Table 4.11 Independent sample test: Price advantages of products marketed by three parallel traders compared to price advantages of products marketed by four and more (Sweden 2003/2004)

	T	df	Sig (1-tailed)	Mean Difference
Different variances assumed	18.2	1 278	0.0000	0.072

The figures presented in Table 4.5 of this chapter suggest that just about five years ago, there was no relation between the average price advantage of a parallel traded product and the number of parallel traders who are simultaneously marketing that product. In 2002, the price gap between parallel traded and locally sourced products was higher in the case of the number of parallel traders being three rather than four or more. In 2003 and 2004, however, we observe that the price difference between locally sourced and parallel traded drugs increases with the number of parallel traders who are marketing that product. From that we conclude that recent reforms concerning the reimbursement and dispensation of products may have triggered an intensification of competition among parallel traders. These reforms are:

• The abolition of a directive to respect a 10 % price gap between the locally sourced and the parallel trader product
  Until the end of the year 2002, parallel traders where requested to respect a minimal price gap of 10%, towards the locally sourced drug. A look at Table 4.5 suggests that in 2001

and 2002 parallel traders would generally set a price which is approximately 10% below the price of the locally sourced product, no matter how many other parallel traders were selling the same product at the same time. From 2003 onwards we observe two trends. Price differences between the locally sourced and the parallel traded product increased for products which are subject to more intense competition and decreased for products which are exposed to less intense competition.

- The generic substitution law in 2002
  The generic substitution law, introduced in 2002, is probably the most important reason why competition among parallel traders has intensified during the last couple of years. Previously, it was good enough to dispense any parallel traded product. From 2002 on, however, pharmacists were requested to always pick the least expensive one. Pharmacists were therefore newly requested to compare prices of all suppliers rather than randomly ordering from one.
- The new ordering system introduced in 2003
  The new ordering system introduced in 2003, highlights the lowest priced of all available interchangeable drugs, whenever the pharmacist enters the brand or the non-proprietary name of a product into the system. If the cheapest supplier has run out of stocks the system automatically proposes the next more expensive product and so forth. The new system helps the pharmacist to dispense the lowest priced alternative at any time. Before its introduction it was possible to order a wrong product by mistake and drive up expenses unconsciously. Especially small parallel traders were at risk of being overlooked by the pharmacists.

4.5.6 The impact of generic and parallel traded competition on the pricing behaviour of drug manufacturers

In the last chapters we have shown that there are situations where the pharmaceutical company can generate higher profits by accommodating parallel trade, rather than by deterring it. Economic theory shows that pharmaceutical companies are more likely to deter if international price differences are low and potential arbitrage volumes large. According to the Swedish and the Norwegian Association of Pharmaceutical Companies, Swedish prices are lower than prices in Denmark. Subsidiaries of pharmaceutical companies in Sweden are, therefore, more likely than these in Denmark to deter parallel trade by setting a price that makes parallel imports unprofitable.

Ganslandt and Maskus were the first to analyse if Swedish prices for locally sourced products respond to parallel traded competition. They found that between 1997 and 1998, prices of locally sourced products in Sweden subject to competition, increased 7.6%, while prices of locally sourced products exposed to parallel traded competition increased by 6.4% only[97]. Competition from parallel trade would have contained price growth of locally sourced pharmaceuticals by 1.2% between 1997 and 1998. In order to verify if the observed difference is statistically significant, Ganslandt and Maskus perform t-tests[98], assuming un-

---

97 M. Ganslandt, K.E. Maskus (2004), J. of Health Economics 23 (2004) 1035–1057, p.1049
98 M. Ganslandt, K.E. Maskus (2004), J. of Health Economics 23 (2004) 1035–1057, p.1049

equal variances, of the hypothesis that the mean change is the same. *"The hypothesis that the manufacturing firms' price changes for goods facing PIs and those not facing such imports is the same, can be rejected at a 5% level for 1997–1998 (t = 1.77), which confirms that the manufacturing firms' prices increased significantly less for products subject to PIs than did prices of other products in the latter part of the period[99]."* When choosing a longer observation period (1994–1998), the hypothesis that price changes for pharmaceuticals which are facing parallel imports are the same as price changes for products not subject to parallel trade cannot be rejected at a 10% level.

Kanavos and Costa-Font[100] find that between 1997 and 2002, prices of originals in Sweden, which were facing no competition at all, decreased by 3%. Prices of originals subject to competition from parallel traded products only decreased by 14% and prices of originals exposed to generic competition decreased by 57%[101]. For Sweden, Kanavos and Costa-Font do not test if the observed differences between the mean price changes of locally sourced products which were or were not exposed to parallel trade, are statistically significant or not. The large difference between the price change of originals which were and were not facing parallel traded competition (11%) is, nevertheless, an indicator that in Sweden, manufacturers of branded products have responded to parallel traded competition by reducing their prices in the time period between 1997 and 2002. Just as the Danish authorities, the LFN began to make use of international reference pricing by the end of the last decade. Government induced price reductions may be a further reason why prices of locally sourced products which are exposed to parallel trade, eased back that strongly between 1997 and 2002.

In order to assert how pharmaceutical companies responded to competition in the course of this decade, we have processed monthly sales information on 196 locally sourced formulations which were available between July 2003 and September 2004. While 91 formulations were not facing any competition during that time period, 63 were subject to competition from parallel traded drugs only and 42 were subject to generic competition[102]. Our evaluation shows that compared to the average price in summer 2003, the average price in summer 2004 was 1.0% lower for branded drugs without competitors, 0.0% lower for branded drugs facing competition from parallel trade only and 9.6% lower for products facing generic competition. Between January 2001 and September 2004, prices of 81 locally sourced products not subject to any competition increased by 0.5% while prices of 56 products exposed to parallel trade only decreased by 0.9%.

In order to assess whether these differences are statistically significant we use t-tests of the hypothesis:

$$H_0 : \mu_A - \mu_B = 0$$

against the alternative

$$H_0 : \mu_A - \mu_B > 0$$

---

99   M. Ganslandt, K.E. Maskus (2004), J. of Health Economics 23 (2004) 1035–1057, p.1049

100   Kanavos P. and Costa-Font J. (2005), Pharmaceutical Trade, Economic Policy October 2005, p. 778

101   Kanavos P. and Costa-Font J. (2005), Pharmaceutical Trade, Economic Policy October 2005, p. 778

102   Own observations based on the 5-year rolling price database from DKMA

at a minimal significance level of $\alpha = 0.05$

with A and B quoting whether products are subject to no, parallel traded or generic competition and μ representing the average price change of a locally sourced product over the time period defined below.

a) Price changes of locally sourced products which were subject to no competition compared to those which were subject to competition from parallel traded products only (2003–2004)

Between 2003 and 2004, prices of locally sourced products, which were not subject to any competition ($\mu_{NO\ Competition}$), decreased by 1.0% ($\sigma_{NO\ Competition} = 0.06008$). In the same time period prices of locally sourced products which are exposed to parallel trade only ($\mu_{PI\ Only}$) have not changed ($\mu_{NO\ Comp} = 0.0$, $\sigma_{PI\ Only} = 0.0$). The number of observations is 92 for products which were not subject to any competition and 63 for products which were exposed to parallel traded competition only. These figures are summarized in Table 4.12.

Table 4.12 Price changes of locally sourced products which were subject to no competition compared to those which were subject to competition from parallel traded products only (Sweden, 2003–2004)

Competitive situation	N° of observations	Unweighted average (μ)	Standard deviation (σ)
No competition	92	−0.00982	0.06008
PI Only	63	0.0	0.0

The Levence's test (F = 8.202, p-value = 0.005) rejects the assumption on the equality of variances. We have therefore run a t-test, assuming *unequal variances,* of the hypothesis sketched above. We find that H_0 cannot be rejected at a 5% level as the test statistic (T = 1.568) is smaller than the critical value for $t_{91;0.05} = 1.66$. However, it is possible to reject H_0 at a 10% significance level. We find some evidence that between 2003 and 2004, prices of locally sourced products which were facing parallel traded competition, have decreased more slowly than prices of locally sourced products which were not facing any competition. By limiting supplies in Southern Europe, originators are able to limit parallel trade volumes. A small increase of the Swedish price would, therefore, have no immediate impact on parallel trade volumes. Pharmaceutical companies may, therefore, decide to increase (or not to reduce) their prices in the destination countries to compensate for the losses they suffer because of parallel trade.

Table 4.13 Independent sample test: Price changes of locally sourced products which were subject to no competition compared to those which were subject to competition from parallel traded products only (Sweden, 2003–2004)

	T	Df	Sig (1-tailed)	Mean Difference
Equal variances assumed	1.568	91	0.0625	−0.00982

b) Price changes of locally sourced products which were subject to no competition compared to those which were subject to competition from parallel traded products only (2001–2004)

Between 2001 and 2004, prices of locally sourced products, which were not subject to any competition ($\mu_{\text{NO Competition}}$), increased by 0.5% ($\sigma_{\text{NO Competition}} = 0.08310$). In the same time period prices of locally sourced products which were exposed to parallel traded competition ($\mu_{\text{PI Only}}$) eased back by 0.9% ($\sigma_{\text{PI Only}} = 0.04985$). The number of observations is 83 for products which were not subject to any competition and 53 for products which were exposed to parallel traded competition only. These figures are summarized in Table 4.14.

The Levence's test ($F = 0.066$, p-value = 0.80) confirms the assumption on the equality of variances. We have therefore run a t-test, assuming *equal variances,* of the hypothesis sketched above. We find that H_0 cannot be rejected at a 5% level as the critical value for $t_{137;0.05} = 1.65$ is larger than the test statistic $T = 1.14$. While H_0 cannot be rejected at a 5% significance level, it is not possible to exclude that, between 2001 and 2004, prices of locally sourced products which are facing parallel traded competition, would have increased more slowly than prices of locally sourced products which were not facing any competition. The minimal significance level at which the hypothesis H_0 could be rejected is 13.1%. All these findings are summarized in Table 4.15.

Table 4.14 Price changes of locally sourced products which were subject to no competition compared to those which were subject to competition from parallel traded products only (Sweden 2001–2004)

Competitive situation	N° of observations	Unweighted average (μ)	Standard deviation (σ)
No competition	83	0.004859	0.08311
PI Only	53	−0.009317	0.04986

Table 4.15 Independent sample test: Price changes of locally sourced products which were subject to no competition compared to those which were subject to competition from parallel traded products only (Sweden 2001–2004)

	T	Df	Sig (1-tailed)	Mean Difference
Equal variances assumed	1.144	137	0.13	0.01418

c) Price changes of locally sourced products which where subject to no competition compared to those which were subject to generic competition (2003–2004)

Between 2003 and 2004, prices of locally sourced products, which were not subject to any competition ($\mu_{\text{NO Competition}}$), decreased by 1.0% ($\sigma_{\text{NO Competition}} = 0.06008$). In the same time period prices of locally sourced products which were exposed to generic competition (μ_{Generic}) decreased by 9.7% ($\sigma_{\text{Generic}} = 0.1492$). The number of observations is 92 for products which were not subject to any competition and 44 for products which were exposed to generic competition. These figures are summarized in Table 4.16.

The Levence's test (F = 69.2, p-value = 0.001) rejects the assumption on the equality of variances. We have therefore run a t-test, assuming *unequal variances,* of the hypothesis sketched above. We find that H_0 can be rejected at a 0.1% level as the critical value for $t_{50;0.001} = 3.26$ is smaller than the test statistic t = 3.718. There is, consequently, strong evidence that pharmaceutical companies respond by cutting their prices as generic competition emerges.

Table 4.16 Price changes of locally sourced products which were subject to no competition compared to those which were subject to generic competition (Sweden 2003–2004)

Competitive situation	N° of observations	Unweighted average (μ)	Standard deviation (σ)
No competition	92	–0.00982	0.06008
Generics	44	–0.09664	0.14919

Table 4.17 Independent sample test: Price changes of locally sourced products which were subject to no competition compared to those which were subject to generic competition (Sweden 2003–2004)

	T	Df	Sig (1-tailed)	Mean Difference
Equal variances assumed	3.718	50	0.0001	0.08682

Ganslandt and Maskus produce significant results (5% level) that between 1997 and 1998 prices of locally sourced, products which were facing parallel traded competition, increased slower than prices of products facing no competition. For the time period between 1994 and 1998, they find that the average price of locally sourced products exposed to parallel trade increased slower than the average price of those exposed to no competition. For the longer observation period, the hypothesis that price changes for both product groups are the same, cannot not be rejected. Kanavos and Costa-Font find that between 1997 and 2002, the average price of a locally sourced product eased back more strongly than the average price of a locally sourced product which is not facing any competition. The LSE economists do not test if the observed difference is significant. It is, nevertheless, possible to assume that between 1997 and 2002, pharmaceutical companies in Sweden responded to parallel traded competition by reducing the Swedish list price. We observe that prices of locally sourced products, which are exposed to parallel trade eased back by 0.9% between 2001 and 2004. In the same period these products facing no competition increased by 0.5%. However, we cannot, at a 10% significance level reject the hypothesis that price changes for goods facing PI and prices changes for goods not facing PI are the same.

Even though statistical significance is not always given overall, the data presented in various publications suggests that parallel traded competition has, over the past twelve years, induced pharmaceutical companies to reduce Swedish list prices. Tests on the significance of observed differences between price changes, respond sensibly to the methodology used, the time frame and the size and composition of the data sample. Concerning the data samples used by different authors we observe that these are generally relatively small. Ganslandt' and Maskus' sample includes 164 forms of 50 molecules[103] and ours 208. The size of the data sample is restricted by the number of molecules which are exposed to parallel trade over an extended period of time and the accessibility to sensitive data. The size of the data samples is therefore one reason why significance of observed differences can often not be confirmed when running statistical tests.

Table 4.18 summarises how, prices of locally sourced drugs responded to parallel traded competition in other destination countries of parallel trade. Figures are taken from Kanavos and Costa-Font[104]. Kanavos and Costa-Font compare price changes between 1997 and 2002 of locally sourced products that are either subject to no, parallel traded or generic competition. They find that prices of locally sourced products not facing competition, decreased quicker (increased slower) than prices of locally sourced products facing parallel traded competition in Denmark, Germany and the Netherlands. These are countries where pharmaceutical companies enjoy a certain degree of freedom of pricing. By practicing supply control in southern Europe, pharmaceutical companies are able to restrict parallel trade volumes. This means that moderate price increases in the destination country, do not necessarily affect parallel trade volumes. It is, therefore, possible that originators have increased domestic prices to compensate for their losses resulting from parallel trade. Evidence from Norway suggests that originators tend to increase their prices after market entry of generic competition[105]. Frank and Salkever come to comparable results when observing prices of 32 pharmaceuticals that lost patent protection during the early 1980s in the US[106]. They observed small price increases on branded pharmaceuticals that became exposed to generic competition.

Kanavos and Costa-Font do not, for the individual country, specify if observed differences are statistically significant. We can, therefore, not say *in confidence* that in Germany, Netherlands and Denmark prices of locally sourced pharmaceuticals exposed to parallel traded competition increased quicker than prices of those not exposed to any competition.

Table 4.18 Relative price change (1997–2002) of locally sourced drugs facing no competition, parallel imported competition only or both, generic and parallel traded competition

	Norway	Denmark	Germany	UK	Sweden	Netherlands
Not facing PI	2%	−13%	2%	N.A.	−3%	4%
Facing PI	1%	−7%	4%	5%	−14%	6%
Facing PI and generic	−30%	−33%	−43%	1%	−57%	−57%

Source: Kanavos P. and Costa-Font J. (2005), Pharmaceutical Trade, Economic Policy October 2005, p. 778

103 M. Ganslandt, K.E. Maskus (2004), J. of Health Economics 23 (2004) 1035–1057, p. 1045

104 Source: Kanavos P. and Costa-Font J. (2005), Pharmaceutical Trade, Economic Policy October 2005, p. 778

105 Dag Morten Dalen et al. (2006), Price regulation and generic competition in the pharmaceutical market, Page 4

106 Frank R.G., Salkever D.S. (1997), "Generic Entry and the Pricing of Pharmaceuticals", J. of Econ & Management Strategy. Spring. pp.75–90

West and Mahon found that parallel trade generated indirect savings in Sweden. For Denmark, they found statistical evidence for competition from parallel imports forcing pharmaceutical manufacturers to lower the prices of the products concerned[107]. However, they reflected that price cuts imposed by the government could be one possible explanation why prices of locally sourced products, which are exposed to parallel trade, eased back more strongly than those which are not exposed to parallel trade.

We conclude that differences between regulatory frameworks and market environments in Sweden and remaining Europe, lead to a different response of pharmaceutical companies which are facing parallel traded competition. Evidence strongly suggests that Swedish subsidiaries of pharmaceutical companies respond to parallel traded competition with moderate price reductions. Apparently, this is not the case in most other European countries. We conclude that Sweden has been more successful in creating a business and regulatory environment that fosters competition than any other destination country of parallel trade. It is therefore not surprising that relative savings from parallel trade are higher in Sweden than in remaining Europe. In the next subsection we summarise what the success factors of the Swedish model are.

4.6   Conclusions for Sweden

Parallel trade in Sweden is generating sizeable savings for consumers and the National Health System. The incentives which are given to patients and pharmacists are highly efficient in generating competition and driving prices of pharmaceuticals down. Sweden's' success, however, is partially based on its distribution system. Indeed, while, pharmacies are privately owned in all other European countries, Sweden maintains its government owned, non-profit pharmacy chain. The distribution system, one of Sweden's success factors, cannot be copied by other countries because it infringes ECJ case law. Below we have listed the four most important success factors of the Swedish policy.

a)   The substitution rule
Pharmacists have been obliged to dispense the cheapest of all chemically identical products since 2002. In order to be able to sell immediately, parallel traders need to offer the lowest price. Parallel traders who charge a higher price for an identical drug than their competitors, are only able to sell once their competitors have emptied their stocks.

b)   The reimbursement system
In Sweden, patients are reimbursed up to the price of the cheapest of all chemically identical products, unless the prescribing physician has excluded generic and parallel traded substitution. Patients who refuse to accept this product are obliged to pay the full price difference out of their own pocket. Furthermore, Sweden has a regressive co-payment system that makes patients with a moderate consumption pay a substantial share of their consumption out of their own pocket. Swedish patients are likely to verify if the product a pharmacist offers, is really the most cost-effective one.

---

107 West P. et al. (2003) Benefits to Payers and Patients From Parallel Trade (2002), The York Health Economics Consortium

c) The electronic pharmacy purchasing system

In 2002, Apoteket AB, the government owned pharmacy chain, introduced a new ordering system. This system pre-selects the lowest priced of all interchangeable products whenever the pharmacist enters a brand or non-proprietary name of a product. It helps pharmacists to identify the cheapest supplier. Pharmacists who intend to order a product other than the one suggested by the ordering system, have to un-tick that specific drug before selecting another one.

d) The government owned monopsonist pharmacy chain

In Sweden, only one government owned pharmacy company is entitled to sell prescription and over the counter drugs to the public. Apoteket AB is a branch of the Ministry of Health which is responsible for setting up, supervising and enforcing the health policy of the Swedish government. Pharmacy tenants receive fixed salaries and no benefits are paid to pharmacists for outperforming the average pharmacy in terms of revenues. The performance of a single pharmacist is not measured in terms of sales but in terms of implementing the saving guidelines which have been defined by the government.

5

Increasing payers benefits
from parallel trade:
Observations from Scandinavia
and policy proposals for Europe

Our case studies from three Scandinavian countries have shown that parallel trade is not lowering drug expenditures to the same extent in all countries. While relative price advantages of parallel traded drugs are sizeable in Sweden, they are very low in Norway.

We have seen that appropriate incentives to patients and the middlemen on one hand and eased market access for parallel traded drugs on the other hand are the key preconditions for effective competition. Parallel trade is more likely to generate considerable savings if:

- Wholesalers and pharmacists have incentives/obligations to dispense the cheapest of all products with the same active substance
- Patients have clear incentives to ask for/purchase the lowest priced product
- Parallel traders enjoy eased market access (i.e. market authorisation is easily granted, if the foreign and the domestic product are (bio)equivalent but not necessarily identical)

On the other hand, savings from parallel trade are likely to remain behind expectations if:

- Patients have no incentives to switch to a lower priced product
- Wholesalers and pharmacists have financial incentives to dispense more expensive products
- Discounts are legal and pharmacists entitled to retain a certain percentage of the discount on a parallel traded drug
- Medicine Control Agencies do not authorize parallel imports if the foreign product version is not identical with the domestic version in terms of
  - Pack size
  - Brand name
  - Formulations (e.g. Losec case in Sweden)

Tables 5.1 and 5.2 provide an overview of how different policies on a wholesaler/ pharmacy/ patient level affect parallel trade volumes and prices.

Over the past thirty years the European Union has removed most internal trade barriers and free movement of goods, services, capital and labour is now a reality. Intra-community trade has led to a price convergence on various fast moving and durable consumer goods. However, the success of the common market should not belie that the convergence process is far from being completed, especially when it comes to pharmaceuticals. The last three chapters have shown that the extent to which prices of pharmaceuticals ease back after a

Table 5.1 Health policies and parallel trade volumes

Level of intervention	Positive	Negative
Medicine Control Agency	• High tolerance towards parallel trade applications with different… – Pack size – Brand name – Formulations (differences are not of therapeutic significance) … compared to the locally sourced drug	• Low tolerance towards parallel trade applications with different … – Pack size – Brand name – Formulations … compared to the locally sourced drug
Wholesaler	• Obligation to contract – Wholesalers are requested to deal with parallel traded drugs • Price-independent remuneration system – Wholesaler margins are not a function of ex-factory prices.	• Freedom to contract – Wholesalers are free to reject parallel imported products • Remuneration is a function of ex-factory prices
Pharmacy	• Dispensation rule • Pharmacies are requested to dispense the lowest priced product • Acquiescence of discounts – Discounts are legal and pharmacies entitled to retain a share of these discounts • Centralized ordering system – Pharmacists are requested to order through a centralized ordering system that pre-selects the lowest priced product • Price-independent remuneration system – Pharmacy margins are not a function of ex-factory prices. Instead pharmacies are remunerated on a per patient/ per pack basis	• Remuneration is a function of ex-factory prices • Freedom of dispensation – Pharmacies have no guidelines concerning the product version they hand out to the patient
Patient	• Reimbursement rule • Multi-tier co-payment plans • High self-contribution	• Flat co-payment • Low self-contribution

trade liberalization, depends on the (dis)incentives wholesaler, pharmacists and patients are given to switch to a lower priced product. The dos and don'ts in healthcare regulation can be derived from Tables 5.1 and 5.2.

Sweden's policy, as we have seen, is very close to the optimal policy that we have sketched above. Whether an optimal environment in the *destination* market is enough to extract all profits from the middlemen, however, still needs to be proven. For that purpose we will, later in this dissertation paper turn our attention to the welfare effects of parallel trade by comparing wholesale prices in source and destination countries.

Table 5.2 Health polices and price advantages of parallel traded products

Level of intervention	Positive	Negative
Wholesaler	• Price-independent remuneration system – Wholesaler margins are not a function of ex-factory prices.	• Remuneration is a function of ex-factory prices

Physician	• Dispensation rule
	• Pharmacies are requested to dispense the lowest priced product
	• Centralized ordering system
	  – Pharmacists are requested to order through a centralized ordering system that pre-selects the lowest priced product
	• Price-independent remuneration system
	  – Pharmacy margins are not a function of ex-factory prices. Instead pharmacies are remunerated on a per patient/ per pack basis
		• Remuneration is a function of ex-factory prices
		• Freedom of dispensation
		• Pharmacies have no guidelines concerning the product version they hand out to the patient
		• Acquiescence of discounts
		  – Discounts are legal and pharmacies entitled to retain a share of these discounts

Patient	• Reimbursement rule • Multi-tier co-payment plans • High self-contribution	• Flat co-payment • Low self-contribution

6

Why do prices not converge?
A theoretical assessment

6.1   Discussion background

Kanavos and Costa-Font contradict the standard arbitrage hypothesis of price competition and the race towards the bottom in the importing countries. They reject the hypothesis of price convergence among exporting and importing countries for Europe as a whole[108]. Evidence from Sweden suggests that pharmaceutical companies respond to parallel traded competition by reducing their list prices, though to a level which is higher than what parallel traders are charging. Price reductions in Sweden may, therefore, have another purpose than *deterring* parallel trade. The reason why pharmaceutical companies reduce their list prices may, nevertheless, be parallel trade.

In this chapter we present a model showing why pharmaceutical companies may be better off by accommodating parallel trade rather than deterring it by reducing the price in the destination country so making parallel trade unprofitable.

6.2   Modelling the realities in pharmaceutical markets

Results by Kanavos and Costa-Font on the price setting behaviour of pharmaceutical companies who are facing parallel traded competition, may be surprising for some. In order to show why drug companies may be indeed better off by accommodating parallel trade rather than deterring it, we have modelled a three country economy.

On the following pages, we present our own model illustrating why pharmaceutical companies may, under certain circumstances, prefer to accommodate parallel trade rather than to deter it by setting the price that makes parallel trade unprofitable. The model is inspired by Ganslandt and Maskus[109]. With the use of this model we show that a pharmaceutical company's decision, whether or not to deter parallel trade, depends on the following circumstances:
- The ratio between the market size of the destination country and the countries which are using the official list price in that destination country as a benchmark

---

108   P. Kanavos, J. Cost Font (2005), Economic Policy October 2005, pp 751–798

109   Ganslandt M and Maskus K (2004): J. of Health Economics 23 (2004) 1035–1057, p.1049 and Ganslandt M and Maskus K (2001): Working Paper No 546, 2001, IUI, Stockholm

- The price gap between the origin and the destination country of parallel trade
- The marginal costs of parallel distribution to the middlemen involved in parallel trade
- The availability of products that can be profitably imported from a low income country.

The assumptions used in our model reflect the regulatory and economic realties in the European Union. Before presenting these assumptions let us – again – look at how EU member countries regulate prices, health expenditures, and supplies.

a) Price regulation
In the European Union, there is not one single country where pricing is completely free. In most European countries, the maximal price that a drug company can charge is set by reference to the lowest or the average price charged in a selection of other countries. If a pharmaceutical company attempts to deter parallel trade by reducing the price in destination country A, pricing authorities in the origin country will insist on having their price reduced too, thus nullifying the effect of having reduced the price in A. Moreover, increasing the price in an origin country of parallel trade is virtually impossible due to price regulations in these countries. Our model aims at illustrating how international reference pricing can void a drug company's effort to deter parallel trade by setting a uniform price.

b) Pharmaceutical budgets
Most governments in Europe are, in one way or another, limiting healthcare and pharmaceutical expenditures. Budgetary control either on a national or on a regional level is currently used by governments of five of the six largest pharmaceutical markets in Europe. Pharmaceutical consumption and pharmaceutical expenditures is therefore a function of budgetary control, rather than one of prices and price elasticity of demand. In our model, we make the assumption, that annual drug expenditures are capped by a pharmaceutical budget. Physicians will always bail out the budget, irrespective of the price of the product.

c) Supply control
In all origin countries of parallel trade, there are regulations concerning the price that a wholesaler may charge to a domestic pharmacy. The price that wholesalers can charge to parallel exporters, however, is often free. From the perspective of a wholesaler, it is, therefore, more attractive to sell a product to a parallel trader who can pay a higher price than the domestic pharmacy. In order to contain parallel exports of pharmaceuticals, drug companies are limiting their supplies to wholesalers in Southern Europe. Supply control has, in the past, led to the situation where wholesalers were unable to respond to domestic demand because they had already sold their products to parallel exporters. This has led to the discussion who should be responsible for securing domestic demand. If pharmaceutical companies alone were responsible for ensuring that pharmacies do not run out of supplies, wholesalers in southern Europe could insist on receiving any quantity that parallel traders are asking for. Theoretically, pharmaceutical companies could end up in the situation where all Europe is supplied from the country where prices are lowest. However, because wholesalers are entrusted, by the government and the pharmaceutical company, to supply domestic pharmacies, it is their duty to ensure that they can – at any time – deliver what the pharmacy is asking for. Wholesalers who are constantly unable to do so because all their supplies have already been sold to a parallel trader may be held liable and are at risk of having their

operation license revoked. Because demand for pharmaceuticals is subject to fluctuations, pharmaceutical companies are requested to supply quantities which are somewhere above anticipated domestic demand. It is because of this, that wholesalers are able to sell some of their products to parallel traders. When it comes to having timely information on domestic demand, wholesalers are in a better position than drug companies. Wholesalers can, therefore, take advantage of that information gap by making drug companies believe that current domestic demand is higher than it effectively is. In our model, we make the assumption that due to regulations and the wholesalers' ability to provide pharmaceutical companies with inaccurate information, the pharmaceutical company will – over the whole year – supply a quantity which is z% above domestic demand of country C. Furthermore we assume that every single pack of pharmaceuticals which has not been used by consumers in C is exported to country A. Our model reflects the situation in Greece, where pharmaceutical companies are requested to provide wholesalers with supplies which are 20% higher than the anticipated domestic demand.

After having explained how prices and supplies are controlled we can present the assumptions of our model:

Let us assume an economy with one low and two high income countries. In that world there is one drug manufacturer selling one universal drug. Annual expenditures on this drug are capped in each of the three countries. Physicians will always bail out the pharmaceutical budget, irrespective of the price of that product[110]. The smaller high income country A passes a law that legalizes parallel imports of pharmaceuticals from country C. Parallel trade in and out of country B is prohibited. Wholesalers and pharmacists in A are requested to dispense the lower priced parallel imported product if such is available. If not, (i.e. parallel traders have run out of stocks) pharmacies are requested to dispense the locally sourced drug.

- Let us assume that prices in these market are regulated as follows:
    - In country A, the pharmaceutical company is free to set any price which is no higher than p_A
    - The price in country B is set as follows by the national pricing authorities:

    $$p_B = \alpha \cdot p_A + (1 - \alpha) \cdot p_C \text{, with } 0 < \alpha < 1$$

    - The price in country C is set as follows by the national pricing authorities:

    $$p_C = \beta \cdot p_A \text{, with } \beta < 1$$

- The pharmaceutical company produces the drug at marginal production costs of mc_P
- The three countries use pharmaceutical budgets B_A, B_B and B_C to limit expenditures on pharmaceutical X.

Parallel traders are able to import products from country C to country A at marginal costs mc_{PD} per unit. Facing shortages of supplies, government C has issued a law that requires the

---

110 Various countries use budgets to cap pharmaceutical expenditures

drug manufacturer to supply a quantity of pharmaceuticals which is z % higher than anticipated domestic demand. Parallel traders are able to source the totality of these excessive supplies and export them to country A.

Let us now look at how changes of z and other basic parameters affect the drug manufacturers' decision whether or not to deter parallel trade by setting a price in A, which makes parallel trading unprofitable.

If parallel trade into country A is prohibited, the pharmaceutical company will charge the market segmentation price in the high revenue country. Units sold and industry profits under market segmentation are described in Functions 6.1 through 6.3

Function 6.1: $\quad q_A = \dfrac{B_A}{p_A}, \quad \pi_A = (p_A - mc_p)\dfrac{B_A}{p_A}$

Function 6.2:

$$q_B = \frac{B_B}{\alpha \cdot p_A + (1 - \alpha)p_A}, \quad \pi_B = ((\alpha \cdot p_A + (1 - \alpha) \cdot p_A) - mc_p)\,\frac{B_B}{\alpha \cdot p_A + (1 - \alpha)p_A}$$

Function 6.3: $\quad q_C = \dfrac{B_C}{\beta \cdot p_A}, \quad \pi_C = (\beta \cdot p_a - mc_p)\dfrac{B_C}{\beta \cdot p_A}$

If country A decides to allow parallel imports from C, the pharmaceutical company has the option between accommodating and deterring them. In order to deter parallel trade, the pharmaceutical company has to lower the price in country A, until the price gap between C and A is equal to marginal costs of parallel distribution. Price reductions in country A lead to immediate price cuts in countries B and C.

Function 6.4 shows that parallel imports can only occur if the price difference between country A and C is larger than marginal costs of parallel distribution. In order to deter parallel trade, the drug company will have to lower p_A until $p_A = mc_{PD}/(1 - \beta)$.

Function 6.4: $\quad mc_{PD} \leq p_A - \beta \cdot p_A \quad \rightarrow \quad p_A = \dfrac{mc_{PD}}{(1 - \beta)}$

After inserting Function 6.4 into Functions 6.1, 6.2 and 6.3, we find that costs of deterring parallel trade (by reference to the situation where these markets are segmented) grow inline with the regulated price gap $(1 - \beta)$ in country C, the relative size of markets B and C compared to market A and the importance of the price in C for the regulator in country B. At the same time, costs of deterring parallel trade diminish with growing marginal costs of parallel distribution.

Accommodating parallel trade, however, is costly too. On every parallel traded pack which is sold in country A, the pharmaceutical company loses the price difference between A and C. If market shares of parallel trade are low, it is reasonable to accommodate parallel trade because losses from having prices cut all over the world are higher than losses from having lower margins on some products which are sold to the end consumer in market A. Let us now look at how the decision of a pharmaceutical company, whether or not to deter parallel trade by lowering prices worldwide, alters as the basic parameters sketched above change. We assume that pharmaceutical expenditures are capped at EUR 50 m in country A, 500 m in country C and 100 m in country B. Government A allows the drug company to set a price of EUR 100, which he will do because his sales are EUR 50 m, no matter what price he sets. By inserting price A in Functions 6.2 and 6.3 we find that the price of the drug is fixed at EUR 95 in country B and EUR 80 in country C. Furthermore we assume that the drug manufacturer has marginal costs of production of EUR 25 and that marginal costs of parallel distribution for bringing the product into country A are EUR 15. All assumptions are summarized in Table 6.1.

Table 6.1 Parameters of the basic model

Price in A (market segmentation)	EUR 100	Budget in A	EUR 50 m
Price in B (Market segmentation)	EUR 95 ($\alpha = 0.75$)	Budget in B	EUR 500 m
Price in C (Market segmentation	EUR 80 ($\beta = 0.8$)	Budget in A	EUR 100 m
Marginal costs of production	25	Marginal costs of parallel distribution	15

Imagine now, that government A decides to allow parallel trade from country C. The pharmaceutical company will now have to decide whether to accommodate or to deter parallel imports from country C.

Let us first look at how the decision to deter parallel trade would affect prices, sales and profits in countries A, B and C. By inserting $mc_{PD} = 15$ and $\beta = 0.8$ into $p_A = mc_{PD} / (1 - \beta)$ we find that the deterrence price p_A is EUR 75. If the drug company decides to set a price of EUR 75 in A pricing authorities in C will insist on having p_C cut to EUR 50 ($p_C = \beta \cdot p_B = 0.8 \cdot 75 = 50$), which is EUR 15 lower than the new p_A. The price regulator in B, would then request that the price for X is reduced to EUR 71.25. Because marginal costs of parallel distribution are EUR 15 too, parallel traders would no longer be able to profitably import the drug into A while setting a price which is lower than p_A.

By inserting budget restrictions and market segmentation and deterrence prices into profit Functions 6.1 through 6.3 we find the following about the cost of deterring parallel trade.

If parallel trade is prohibited and drug companies able to set the market segmentation price in A, B and C, *global profits* of the drug company are EUR 474.7 m. If parallel trade is legal and the drug company decides to set the deterrence price his global profits are EUR 416.2 m. Setting the deterrence price will, therefore, cost the drug company EUR 58.4 m, compared to the situation where parallel trade is prohibited and the drug company is able to set the market segmentation prices in A, B and C. A closer view at Table 6.2 reveals that 92% of the losses resulting from deterring parallel trade occur in countries B and C. Moreover, losses from deterring parallel trade (EUR 58.4 m) are higher than profits in country A under market segmentation (EUR 37.5 m).

Table 6.2 Pricing, sales and profits under market segmentation and deterrence of parallel trade

Market segmentation	Sales (m EUR)	Price EUR	Units sold (.000)	Profits (m EUR)
Country A	50	100.0	500.0	37.5
Country B	500	95.0	5 263.1	368.4
Country C	100	80.0	1 250.0	68.8
World	*650*	*92.7*	*7 913.1*	*474.7*
Deterrence	Sales (m EUR)	Price EUR	Units sold (.000)	Profits (m EUR)
Country A	50	75.0	666.7	33.3
Country B	500	71.2	7 017.5	324.6
Country C	100	60.0	1 666.7	58.3
World	*650*	*69.5*	*9 350.9*	*416.2*
Impact of trade liberalization if deterrence strategy is chosen	Sales	Price	Units sold	Profits
Absolute	+0	−23.2	2 337.8	−58.4
Relative	+0%	−25.0%	33.3%	−12.3%

Instead of deterring parallel trade by cutting his prices in A, B and C, the pharmaceutical company may also decide to maintain $p_A = 100$, $p_B = 95$ and $p_C = 80$ and allow parallel trade to happen.

If the company decides to accommodate parallel trade, all products in countries B and C will keep selling at $p_B = 95$ and $p_C = 80$. Profits from selling pharmaceuticals to consumers in B and C will be the same as under market segmentation. In country A, however, there will now be two types of products: the locally sourced product that will sell at the price of $p_A = 100$ and the parallel traded product that will sell at price of p_{PI}. Industry profits in country A will now be a function of the number of locally sourced and parallel traded products sold in A and the budget restriction imposed by government A. Industry profits and the budget restriction in A are described in Functions 6.5 and 6.6.

Function 6.5: $\pi_A = q_A \, (p_A - mc_p) + q_{PI} \, (p_C - mc_p)$

Function 6.6: $B_A = q_A \cdot p_A + q_{PI} \cdot p_{PI}$

Assuming perfect competition among parallel traders, we can expect them to sell their products at marginal costs of procurement and parallel distribution which, in the given example, is EUR 95 (Procurement price in country C is EUR 80 and marginal costs of parallel distribution is EUR 15). If parallel traders held a market share of 100%, the number of packs sold to consumers in A would be 526 315. Inserting $q_A = 0$ and $q_{PI} = 526 315$ into Functions 6.2, 6.3 and 6.5 yields to $\pi_A = 28.9$ m and to global profits of EUR 466.3 m. No matter what the market penetration of parallel traded products in A is, accommodating parallel trade will always lead to higher profits than setting the deterrence price.

We have now shown, that under the model assumptions which are sketched above, accommodating parallel trade is always better than deterring it, no matter what the market shares of parallel imported products in A are. A glance at Table 6.2 shows that 92% of the losses resulting from deterring parallel trade occur in countries B and C. By how much the drug manufacturer needs to reduce the price in A, so that $p_A - p_B = (1-\beta)\cdot p_A < mc_{PD}$ and parallel trade is no longer profitable, depends on β. The extent, to which the price cuts in countries A and C affect the price in country B, $p_B = \alpha\cdot p_A + (1-\alpha)\cdot p_C$ depends on α. The more important the price of country C in country B's pricing function, the bigger the price cut in B, resulting from reducing the price in A. Costs of deterring parallel trade are, therefore, a negative function of α and β. The larger markets B and C are compared to A, the higher the costs of deterring parallel trade. The question shall therefore be, by how much do we need to increase α and β/reduce the relative size of countries B and C compared to A, until deterring parallel trade becomes an option from the perspective of the pharmaceutical company?

Leaving the other factors unchanged, we increase β from 80 to 84.5%. Given $\beta = 84.5\%$ the manufacturer can deter parallel trade by setting p_A to EUR 96.8. Pricing authorities in C would then ask the manufacturer to set a price of EUR 81.8 (from $p_C = \beta\cdot p_A = 0.845\times 96.8$) while authorities in B would insist on receiving a price of EUR 93. With, $p_A - p_C = 15$, parallel traders are no longer capable to import the product into country A without suffering losses, while setting a price which is lower than what the drug manufacturer is asking for.

By inserting $p_A = 96.8$, $p_B = 93$, and $p_C = 81.8$ into profit Functions 6.1, 6.2 and 6.3 we find that the drug manufacturer would generate profits of EUR 472 m when deterring parallel trade, which is just about EUR 5.7 m less than what he could earn if markets where segmented. Imagine now, that the pharmaceutical company decides to accommodate parallel trade and that competition among parallel traders is perfect. The price of parallel imported product sold in C would then be $p_{PI} = p_C + mc_{PD} = 84.5 + 15 = 99.5$. Given $B_A = 50\cdot 10^6$ and $p_{PI} = 99.5$ the maximal number of parallel traded packs that can possibly be sold in A is 502 512. The number of locally sourced products sold in A would then be zero, due to the budget restriction. Inserting $q_A = 0$ and $q_{PI} = 502512$ into Function 6.5 yields to $\pi_A = 29.9$ m and global profits of EUR 466.9 m. Because minimal profits from accommodating parallel trade (EUR 466.9 m) are lower than profits under deterrence (EUR 472 m), there are situations when deterrence leads to higher profits than accommodation.

The question that the drug manufacturer will have to ask is therefore: "Under which combination of $B_A = q_A\cdot p_A + q_{PI}\cdot p_{PI}$ are global profits from deterring parallel trade identical to global profits from accommodating parallel trade?"

Above we have seen that, when setting the deterrence prices $p_A = 96.8$, $p_B = 93$, and $p_C = 81.8$, global profits are EUR 5.7 m lower than when setting the segmentation prices $p_A = 100$, $p_B = 95$, and $p_C = 80$ and parallel trade is prohibited. Moreover, the decision to accommodate parallel trade affects profits in country A only.

Knowing that profits under deterrence are EUR 5.7 m lower than under market segmentation and a decision to accommodate does affect profits in market A only, the drug manufacturer has to seek for the combination of q_A and q_B where:

Function 6.7: $\pi_{A, \text{Acommodate}} = \pi_{A, \text{Market Segmentation}} - (\Pi_{\text{Global, Market Segmentation}} - \Pi_{\text{Global, Deterrence}})$.

To assert under which q_A and q_B the relation described in Function 6.7 is met, we proceed by inserting the pricing and budget restrictions into Functions 6.8 and 6.9, which are described hereafter.

Function 6.8 describes the industry profits from all locally sourced and parallel traded products sold in A. Whenever a locally sourced product is sold in A, the drug manufacturer generates a profit margin of EUR 75 ($m_A = p_A - mc_P = 100 - 25 = 75$). Whenever a parallel traded drug is sold in A, the drug manufacturer generates a profit margin of EUR 59.5 ($m_A = p_A - mc_P = 84.5 - 25 = 59.5$). Knowing that $\pi_{A, \text{Market Segmentation}} = 37.5\,m$ and that ($\Pi_{\text{Global, Market Segmentation}} - \Pi_{\text{Global, Deterrence}}) = 5.7\,m$ we have to find out under which q_A and q_B, $\pi_{A, \text{Acommodate}} = 37.5\,m - 5.7\,m = 31.8\,m$.

Function 6.8:

$\pi_{A, \text{Acommodate}} = q_A\,(p_A - mc) + q_{PI}\,(p_C - mc) \quad \longleftrightarrow \quad 31.8 \cdot 106 = q_A \cdot 75 + q_{PI} \cdot 59.5$

Function 6.9 describes the combined expenditures on all locally sourced and parallel traded pharmaceuticals sold in A. The pharmaceutical budget of A restricts drug expenditures to EUR 50 m. Physicians will always bail out that budget no matter what the price of the products sold in A are. The price of the locally sourced product is EUR 100. The lowest price that a parallel trader can charge without making losses is EUR 99.5, which is the sum of the purchasing price in C and transaction costs of bringing the product into A (84.5 + 15). Assuming that competition has driven the price of the parallel traded drug down to marginal costs of procurement and distribution we can, therefore, describe a budget restriction as written in Function 6.9.

Function 6.9: $B_A = q_A \cdot p_A + q_{PI} \cdot p_{PI} \quad \longleftrightarrow \quad 50 \cdot 10^6 = q_A \cdot 100 + q_{PI} \cdot 99.5$

By resolving Functions 6.8 and 6.9 we find that market shares of parallel traded products have to grow to 75.6% before deterrence becomes the optimal strategy. In order to enable parallel traders to reach such market shares, supplies in country C would need to be 32.1% above domestic demand. Table 6.3 shows that profits in A are 31.8 m when the number of locally sourced packs sold is 122 500 and the number of parallel traded products is 379 300. In this case only 24.4% of all products sold in A are locally sourced.

Table 6.3 Sales and profits of locally sourced and parallel traded drugs

	Locally sourced	Parallel imported	Overall
Units Sold ('000)	122.5	379.3	501.9
Sales (m EUR)	12.2	37.7	50.0
Profits (m EUR)	9.2	22.6	31.8
Units sold (% of total)	24.4%	75.6%	100%
Sales (% of total)	24.5%	75.5%	100%
Profits(% of total)	28.9%	71.1%	100%

We have now seen that the pricing schemes in third countries are an important factor in determining whether or not a drug manufacturer should deter parallel trade, *by setting the price that makes parallel trade unprofitable.* Manufacturers are more likely to deter the smaller the spill-over effect of cutting back prices in the destination country of parallel trade is on the price level in other countries.

In order to illustrate how an increase of α and β, a decrease of marginal costs of parallel distribution or a decrease of the pharmaceutical budget in countries B and C affect the drug manufacturers decision when to deter, we have entered the respective parameters into Functions 6.7 through 6.9.

Table 6.4 shows that when β is 84.5% and the pharmaceutical budget in countries B and C is EUR 250 m and 75 m respectively, supplies in C have to be 24.8% above domestic demand before deterring parallel trade becomes profitable. If marginal costs of parallel trade fall to EUR 12, the pharmaceutical company would not, under any circumstances, deter parallel trade. Losses from reducing prices in A, B and C would in any case be higher than giving up the entire market A to parallel traders.

Table 6.4 Supplies needed – as a percentage of demand in C – to make the pharmaceutical company deter

Alternative scenario	$(1 - \beta)$	15.5%	16.0%	17.5%	20.0%
Basic model		32.1%	never	never	never
Marginal costs of parallel distribution = 12		never	never	never	never
$\alpha = 0.5$		33.1%	never	never	never
Budget in countries B (250 m) and C (75 m)		24.8%	48.9%	never	never

6.3   Implications

The model has shown that because of international reference pricing by governments, a decision to reduce the price in one country has a considerable impact on prices and profits in other countries. International reference pricing is, therefore, undermining competition between pharmaceutical companies and parallel traders. The concept of taking account of what drug companies charge in other countries is relatively new. By the beginning of the 1990s, not one European country had implemented a system of international benchmarking. Today, there are only two western European countries where pricing authorities do not take reference towards foreign prices.

A recent survey by the consultancy firm IMS health shows that in Europe, the average gap between the highest and the lowest *launch* price is narrowing. Their analysis on 50 recent product launches in 16 countries shows that in 1997, the average difference between the highest and the lowest launch price was 50% compared to just 20% in 2002[111]. IMS health

---

111   Cambridge Pharma Consultancy (2006), Pricing and Market Access Review, p. 8

concludes that this trend is the consequence of governments benchmarking foreign against domestic prices, the difficulties to obtain price premiums in the United Kingdom and Germany and pharmaceutical companies trying to avoid parallel trade.

We conclude that once a product has been launched, pharmaceutical companies are unlikely to adapt prices in the origin and destination country to an extent that makes parallel trade unprofitable. Before launching a product, however, pharmaceutical companies will seek to narrow price differences in northern and southern Europe to an extent that makes parallel trade unprofitable. This, however, does not necessarily mean that the observed convergence of launch prices is beneficial to consumers.

First, there is strong evidence that increased pressure from parallel trade goes hand in hand with longer market access delays in Southern Europe. Table 6.5 shows market access delays of products launched between January 1997 and June 2001 compared these launched between June 2000 and June 2004. We see that market access delays experienced considerable increases in the four most important origin countries of parallel trade. Second, the trend towards smaller launch price gaps does not necessarily imply that average launch prices are falling, which would be a precondition for a positive welfare effect.

Table 6.5 Average time delay between market authorisation and effective market access

	January 1997–June 2001	June 2000–2004	Change 97/01–00/04
Greece	355	427	+20%
France	389	431	+10%
Italy	208	345	+66%
Spain	161	327	+103%

Source: Cambridge Pharma Consultancy (2006)

We summarize that international benchmarking and parallel trade leads to a convergence of launch prices. However, the average time delay between market authorisation and effective market access is on the rise in the most typical origin countries of parallel trade. Whether the net welfare effect is positive or negative requires further evaluation. Once a product has been launched, pharmaceutical companies are often inclined to accommodate parallel trade rather than deterring it by reducing the price in the destination countries to a level that makes parallel trade unprofitable. It is, nevertheless, possible that pharmaceutical companies grant minor price reductions on products which are exposed to parallel trade provided that price reductions granted to consumers in the destination country do not spill over to other countries. It is also possible that pharmaceutical companies may try to compensate for their losses resulting from parallel trade by increasing the list price of products affected by parallel trade. Pharmaceutical companies can do so because supplies in Southern Europe are limited. A moderate price increase in the destination country may not necessarily increase parallel trade volumes.

6.4   Summary

Prices of pharmaceuticals are subject to regulations. These price regulations have a significant influence on a pharmaceutical company's decision on how to reply to parallel trade. This model shows that government interventions such as international reference pricing, reduce a drug company's incentive to deter parallel trade. By practicing supply control, pharmaceutical companies can limit their losses resulting from parallel trade. Practicing supply control and allowing some parallel trade to happen is seen as a profitable alternative to the option of setting a uniform price in Europe.

7

Welfare effects of parallel trade

7.1   Discussion background

Opponents to parallel trade claim that it is highly inefficient and that savings to the consumers are only a fraction of the profits to the middlemen. Advocates oppose that savings to the consumers are high and profit margins of parallel traders low. This chapter looks at evidence on consumer gains and parallel distribution mark ups from the past decade. It shows how these figures have evolved over time and draws conclusions on the future development of the ratio between parallel distribution mark-ups and consumer gains.

7.2   A summary of past research

During the past decade, various studies have addressed the question on the savings resulting from parallel trade in Europe. Only three of them, however, have asked how the price difference between the factory gate in the origin countries and the pharmacy shelf in the destination market is split between the various actors involved in parallel trade.

The oldest study, presented by the London based consultancy firm NERA, used pricing information on parallel traded and locally sourced products in the principal destination and origin countries of parallel trade. Data was provided to NERA by nine leading drug companies in Europe. Each company was requested to submit information on its five most parallel traded products.

NERA finds that in 1996, the average parallel traded drug was priced 22% below the locally sourced drug. For products which are exposed to parallel trade, the average spread between the wholesaler price in the origin and the destination country was 115%. The parallel distribution mark-up was 68%[112]. According to NERA's estimates 60% of the spread between the official list price in the origin and the destination country go to the middlemen, leaving 40% to the patient. These are averages for Denmark, Germany, the Netherlands and the United Kingdom.

In 2005, Kanavos and Costa-Font, presented estimates on savings and welfare effects from parallel traded pharmaceuticals in Denmark, Germany, Norway, The Netherlands, Sweden and the United Kingdom. By using pricing information on 19 top selling products, the authors find that the average parallel imported product is 15.8% cheaper than the locally sourced product in the Netherlands, compared to 8.4% in Denmark, 6.7% in Germany, 2.5%

112   Glynn D. et al. (1997), Survey of parallel trade, Pages 8, 16

Norway and 0.0% in the United Kingdom[113]. The value for the UK is misleading because in Britain, it is the policy to set a fixed list price and to offer discounts rather than reducing list prices as competition emerges. Every year, pharmacies are requested to reimburse a specific share of their revenues to the NHS. That *"claw-back"*, as it is called, reflects the discounts that pharmacies have collected during the past year. In 2003 the pharmacy claw-back was 10.3%. Lacking information on what the NHS knows about discounts granted by parallel traders, the authors use that 10.3% gap as a proxy for the average price difference between locally sourced and parallel traded products. When taking account of the *claw-back* in the UK and the Netherlands, the average parallel traded pack in Europe was priced 7.2% below the locally sourced pack.

Besides presenting estimates on the net savings from parallel trade, Kanavos and Cost-Font have also addressed the welfare issue of parallel trade. By comparing wholesaler prices in southern and northern Europe, they find that 13.4% of the difference between the official wholesaler price in these regions go to the patient while 86.4% are retained by the middle-men. The share of the price spread between the origin and the destination country that goes to the consumer is highest in the Netherlands (30.7%) and lowest in Norway (6.1%). The parallel distribution mark-up for the four countries which were covered by NERA was 47%. Table 7.1 summarises the results which we have presented in the last two paragraphs and provides some further details on savings and welfare effects of parallel trade in Europe's most important destination markets.

Kanavos and Costa-Font and NERA present estimates on the average parallel distribution mark-up for a selection of products. The parallel distribution mark-up is determined by calculating the spread between the wholesaler price of a parallel traded drug in the destination country and the official wholesaler price of the product in the origin country. This parallel distribution mark-up is split between a number of middlemen including the wholesaler or a hospital in the origin country, the parallel importer and the wholesaler in the destination country. Based on the figures presented by Kanavos and Costa-Font, we cannot tell how that parallel distribution mark-up is split between the different middlemen involved in parallel trade. A recent study by Pedersen[114] addresses the question, by showing that an important share of the parallel distribution mark-up is collected by parallel exporters (wholesalers, pharmacies and hospitals in the origin countries) and pharmacists in the destination country. Parallel importers, however, are only accountable for a small share of the parallel distribution margin.

Pedersen uses information on prices at different levels of the supply chain for a selection of high revenue products and finds that the parallel *importer's* mark up, which is the ratio between the price that the parallel trader charges to a wholesaler in the destination country and the price that he pays to his suppliers in the origin country is 13% in Sweden and 22% in Denmark, as shown in Table 7.2.

From the figures presented by Pedersen, we derive that the share of the difference between the ex-factory price in the origin and the wholesaler price in the destination country

113 Kanavos P. and Costa-Font J (2005), Pharmaceutical parallel trade in Europe: stakeholder and competition effects, Economic Policy October 2005, p 778

114 Pedersen K. et al. (2006), The Economic Impact of parallel import of pharmaceuticals, University of Southern Denmark

Table 7.1 Aggregate net benefits from pharmaceutical parallel trade on stakeholders (in m EUR) 2002

	DE	UK	NL	SE	DK	NO	All EUR
Total sales all pharmaceuticals	2 208.3	1 972.3	534.9	535.7	138.7	196.4	5 576
Market penetration parallel imported drugs	18.3%	27.4%	19.0%	31.0%	28.1%	18.3%	25.0%
Price spread PI/ locally sourced drugs	6.7%	10.3%[a]	15.8%	2.2%	8.4%	2.5%	7.2%[b]
Savings from parallel imported drugs	17.7	55.9	19.1	3.8	3.0	0.8	100.3
Parallel distributor revenues	98.0	469.9	43.2	18.4	7.4	12.4	649.3
Maximal savings potential from parallel trade[c]	115.7	535.8	62.3	22.2	10.4	13.2	749.6
Consumer share on international price gap	15.3%	10.6%	30.7%	17.1%	28.9%	6.1%	13.4%
Share of parallel distributors in int. price gap	84.7%	89.4%	69.3%	82.9%	71.1%	94.9%	86.6%

[a] Including the effect of the claw-back. In the UK these are estimates only
[b] Own calculations based on Kanavos P. and Costa-Font J (2005), Economic Policy October 2005, p 778
[c] Assuming that parallel imported products sell at the foreign ex-factory price
Source: Kanavos P. and Costa-Font J (2005), Pharmaceutical parallel trade in Europe: stakeholder and competition effects, Economic Policy October 2005, p 778

which is added by the *importer* is approximately 20% in Denmark and close to 50% in Sweden. While these are rough estimates, we can say, that a substantial share of the difference between the ex-factory price in the origin country and the pharmacy purchasing price for the parallel traded product in the destination country is added by traditional wholesalers in the origin country. In order to bring parallel distribution mark-ups down and to drive consumer savings up, policy reforms are therefore necessary in both the origin and the destination countries of parallel trade.

Substantial share of the difference between the ex-factory price in the origin country and the pharmacy purchasing price for the parallel traded product in the destination country is added by traditional wholesalers in the origin country. In order to bring parallel distribution mark-ups down and to drive consumer savings up, policy reforms are therefore necessary in both the origin and the destination countries of parallel trade.

Table 7.2 Breaking up the parallel distribution mark-ups in Denmark and Sweden

	Sweden	Denmark
Price difference between parallel traded and locally sourced products	15%	7.4%
Parallel *importer's* mark-up	13%	22%
Share of the difference between the ex-factory price in the origin and the wholesaler price in the destination country added by the exporter (i.e. wholesalers, pharmacies etc. in origin country)	50%	80%
Share of the difference between the ex-factory price in the origin and wholesaler price in the destination country added by the importer	50%	20%

Source: Own compilation based on: Pedersen K. et al. (2006), The Economic Impact of parallel import of pharmaceuticals, University of Southern Denmark

7.3 Asserting the welfare effects of parallel trade in Sweden and Denmark

We will now present new estimates on the efficiency of the parallel distribution chain in Sweden and Denmark. We use pricing information on 25 products in Greece, France, Spain, Sweden and Denmark. The French dataset provides information on the ex-factory prices of all products effective in 2005. We calculate the French wholesaler price by multiplying the ex-factory price with the respective wholesaler mark-up. The Greek dataset shows retail prices for all products effective as of January 1st, 2005. We calculate wholesaler prices by deducting VAT and the pharmacy mark up from the retail price. The Spanish dataset shows the ex-factory and the retail price as effective in 2005. We calculate the Spanish wholesaler price by multiplying ex-factory prices with the respective wholesaler mark-up. For Sweden we use wholesaler prices for locally sourced and parallel traded products as effective in June 2005. For Denmark we use wholesaler prices for locally sourced and parallel traded products as effective in the first two quarters of 2005. To convert Danish prices into Euros we used the six month exchange rate (Jan 05- Jun 05) as published on the webpage of the European Central Bank[115]. To convert Swedish prices into Euro we use the exchange rate as effective in June 2005[116].

In order to assert how the price difference between the locally sourced product in the origin and the destination market is split between parallel traders and consumers, we compare wholesaler prices of locally sourced and parallel traded drugs in the two countries. The rationale behind comparing wholesaler prices instead of ex-factory prices is the following. Drug manufacturers have no obligation to supply parallel traders directly. Instead, parallel traders buy their products from wholesalers, pharmacists and hospitals in the low price country. Figure 7.1 illustrates the classical and a parallel distribution chain. In this particular

---

115   1 EUR = 6.44 DKK
116   1 EUR = 9,26 SEK

case, wholesalers in southern Europe sell their products to a parallel trader, rather than to community pharmacists in their own country. Parallel traded products are then supplied to regular wholesalers in the destination country. Compared to the classical, the parallel distribution chain involves two additional middlemen. The parallel distribution mark-up corresponds to the mark-up which is added by the parallel trader and the domestic wholesaler.

Figure 7.1 The classical and the parallel distribution chain in Sweden and Denmark

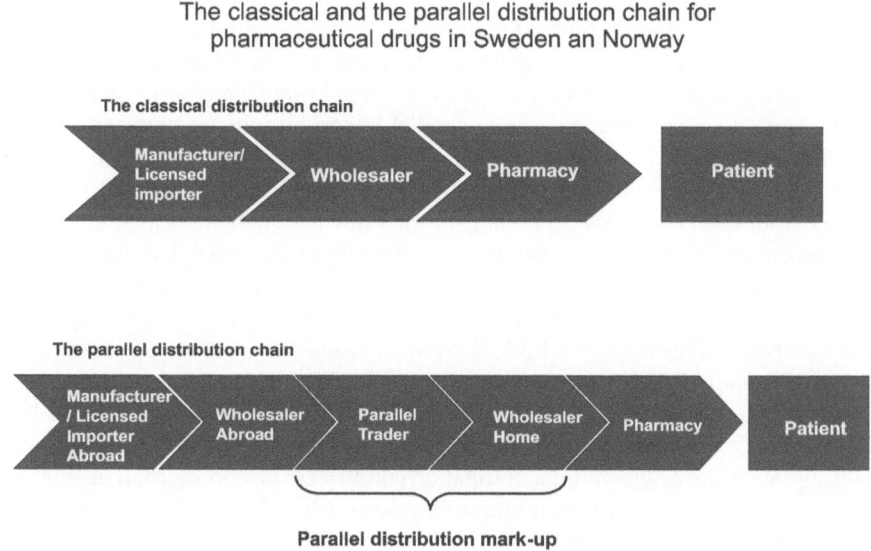

In practice, the parallel distribution chain is often longer than illustrated in Figure 7.1. Often parallel traders buy their products from hospitals or pharmacists who charge more than the official wholesaler price. In Spain, wholesalers are charging higher prices to parallel traders than to community pharmacies. However, because these prices are kept confidential by the business partners, we are not able to tell, which share of the parallel distribution mark-up is added by foreign suppliers, parallel traders and domestic wholesalers.

7.4   The situation in Denmark

In Denmark, the price that a wholesaler or parallel trader may charge to a pharmacist for a specific product is published and updated fortnightly on the website of the Danish Medicine Agency. The Database does not contain any information on the number of parallel traded units sold. Neither does it tell us from which country the parallel imported packs originated. We can therefore only make assumptions on the welfare effect of parallel trade using different scenarios.

The first scenario assumes that every parallel traded pack which is marketed in Denmark originates from the southern European country where prices are the lowest and that Danish consumers buy from the cheapest parallel trader only. The second scenario assumes that France, Greece and Spain supply one third of all parallel traded packs each and sales are split equally among parallel importers active in Denmark. The third scenario assumes that France, Greece and Spain supply one third of all parallel traded packs each and that Danish consumers buy from the cheapest parallel trader only.

For all three calculation methods we use the domestic wholesaler price for the locally sourced drug. The difference between the official list price in southern Europe and the price for the parallel traded good in Denmark is a proxy for wholesaler gains. The difference between the price for the locally sourced and the parallel traded good in Denmark is a proxy for consumer gains. The ratio between wholesaler gains and the international price gap for locally sourced products, is an indicator for the costs of bringing a pharmaceutical to Denmark, the intensity of competition among parallel traders and the efficiency of the parallel distribution chain. Table 7.3 gives an overview of the results from Denmark.

Table 7.3 shows that consumer gains, as a percentage of the international price difference range from 18.5% to 20.8% depending on what calculation method we use. Wholesaler gains as percentage of the price spread between the official pharmacy purchasing price for the locally sourced product in the origin and the destination country range from 79.2% to 81.5%. The parallel distribution margin is in the range between 34.9% and 41.7%.

A comparison of figures from NERA, Kanavos & Costa-Font and us suggests that parallel distribution mark-ups have eased back considerably over the past ten years. In the same time, international price differences of products which are exposed to parallel trade have eased back too. For that reason, consumer savings as a percentage of the spread between the official list price in the origin and the destination country are now lower than in 1996. What the data suggest is that competition and a narrowing price range between northern and southern Europe have driven parallel distribution margins down.

Table 7.3 Parallel distribution mark-ups Denmark

Calculation model		Consumer gains % of price difference	Wholesaler gains % of price difference	Parallel distribution mark-up
1	Average	18.5%	81.5%	41.7%
	Lowest	1.9%	46.2%	11.1%
	Highest	53.8%	98.1%	258.6%
2	Average	19.7%	80.3%	34.9%
	Lowest	2.2%	35.7%	6.1%
	Highest	64.3%	97.8%	258.6%
3	Average	20.8%	79.2%	36.3%
	Lowest	2.2%	35.6%	6.0%
	Highest	64.4%	97.8%	258.6%

Sources: Own calculations based on LIFDK & LIF

Figure 7.2 The relationship between international price gap and parallel distribution mark-up in Denmark

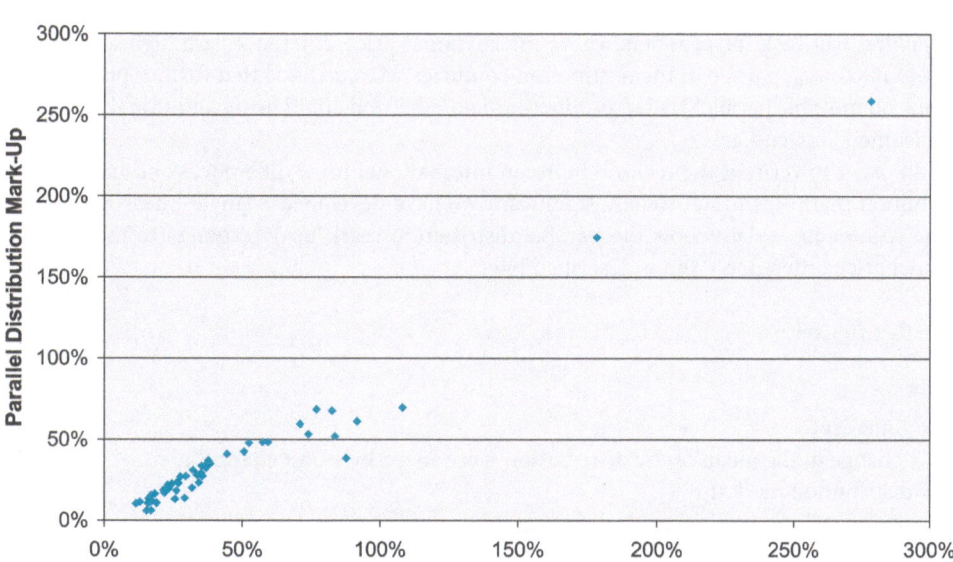

We will now address the question of whether Danish consumers are exploiting the maximum savings potential from parallel trade already or if further price reductions could be achieved by taking the right measures.

A look at the profit and loss statement of Orifarm, Scandinavia's largest parallel trader, shows that in 2005, the corporation's return on revenues was 1.5% only[117]. Provided that Orifarm is making efficient use of its resources, payments to the company owners or the executive team are not excessive and the company is representative for the entire industry, we could conclude that parallel distributors are already operating at marginal costs of parallel distribution. This would imply that further price reductions by parallel traders are not possible. In the long run, we could expect parallel traders to set prices which are about 10% below the price of the locally sourced product.

To verify the plausibility of this interpretation, we test for a relation between parallel distribution mark-ups and international price differences. If no such relation exists it is possible that the parallel distribution chain is operating at marginal costs already. If there is a positive relation, however, further savings can be achieved from parallel trade, even without increasing volumes.

Figure 7.2 shows that there is indeed a strong relation between parallel distribution mark-ups and international price differences. This implies that prices of parallel traded products are set by reference to the Danish, rather than by the southern European list price. A further look at the dataset shows that parallel distribution mark ups vary considerably, not only

---

117 http://www.orifarm.dk/sw5889.asp, Accessed 18.04.2007

in relative, but – more importantly – in absolute terms. While in 2005 the lowest parallel distribution mark up was just about EUR 1.94, the highest mark up was more than forty times higher, namely EUR 78.95. The latter example shows that parallel traders, *and their suppliers,* will seek for products where international price differences are high and set the profit maximising price in the destination countries. We conclude that further price reductions on multiple parallel traded products are possible and could bring additional savings to consumers in Denmark.

In order to verify if the relation between international price differences and parallel distribution mark ups is statistically significant we have developed a single linear regression. The regression explains how the parallel distribution mark-up y responds to the international price difference x and is described by

$$y = \beta_0 + \beta_1 \cdot x + \varepsilon$$

with
β_0 = intercept
β_1 = change in the mean of the distribution y produced by a unit change in x
y = distribution mark up
x = regressor international price difference
ε = random error

The SPSS regression output shows that a 1% increase of the international price difference leads to a 0.89% increase of the parallel distribution mark-up. The regression's intercept is –0.038. We can therefore describe the relation between the international price difference and the parallel distribution mark up of a product which is brought into Sweden by the following function.

$$y = -0.038 + 0.89\, x + \varepsilon$$

Table 7.4 Regression analysis relation between distribution mark-ups and price differentials Denmark

Regression analysis					
Predictor	**Coef.**	**St. Dev**	**T**	**P**	
Constant	−0.0375		−2.20	0.031	
International price difference	0.894		33.311	0.001	
	R-sq	0.956	**R-sq (adj.)**	0.955	
Analysis of variance					
Source	**DF**	**SS**	**MS**	**F**	**P**
Regression	1	8.307	8.307	1.109	0.000
Error	51	0.382	0.007		
Total	52	8.689			

Source: Own calculations, based on the national pricing authorities' data in Europe

The statistical t-value for the slope (33.3) is larger than the critical t-value for a significance level of 1% $t_{51;0.005} = 2.68$, meaning that we can, at a 1% significance level, say that there is a linear relationship between y and x. The statistical t-value for the intercept (–2.2) is larger than the critical t-value for a significance level of 5% $t_{51;0.025} = 2.1$. An analysis of the variance of the regression shows that we can, at a 1% level, reject the hypothesis that β_0 and $\beta_1 = 0$ since the critical F-value $F_{0.01,1,51} = 7.2$ is smaller than the statistical F value (1.109). With 95.6% of the variation being explained by the regressor x we can say in confidence that the regression provides a solid explanation for the relation between international price differences and parallel distribution mark-ups. These findings confirm that prices of parallel traded products are set by reference to the list price in Denmark rather than by reference to the price in the origin country of parallel trade. The findings that we have described above are listed in Table 7.4.

7.5   The situation in Sweden

In Sweden, prices that wholesalers may charge for specific products are published on the website of the Pharmaceutical Benefits Board (LFN). Prices are grouped by product, dosage, pack size, and importer/manufacturer. The database does not contain any information on the number of parallel traded units sold. Neither does it tell us from which country the parallel imported packs originate. We can therefore only make assumptions on the welfare effect of parallel trade using the same scenarios as in the case of Denmark. Table 7.5 gives an overview of the results from Sweden. It shows that parallel distribution mark-ups and wholesaler gains as a percentage of the international price difference are lower in Sweden than in Denmark. This is unsurprising because savings form parallel trade are higher in Sweden than in Denmark too.

Table 7.5 shows that consumer gains, as percentage of the international price difference range from 28.3% to 36.3% depending on which calculation method we use. Wholesaler gains as a percentage of the international price difference range from 63.7% to 71.7%. The parallel distribution margin is in the band between 28.3% and 35.2%.

Our data shows that Swedish patients are getting a larger share of the difference between the official list price in the origin and the destination country when buying a parallel traded product, than patients in Denmark. This, however, does not mean that consumer savings could not be any higher. Let us therefore once more see if there is a relation between international price differences and parallel distribution mark-ups. Our dataset shows that parallel distribution mark ups vary considerably not only in relative, but – much more important – in absolute terms. In 2005 the lowest parallel distribution mark up was 20 cents. The highest mark up, however, was over 500 times higher, namely EUR 135. The latter example shows that parallel traders and their suppliers will seek for products where international price difference are high and set the profit maximising price in the destination countries.

In order to verify if the relation between international price differences and parallel distribution mark ups is statistically significant, we have developed a single linear regression. The regression explains how the parallel distribution mark-up y responds to the international price difference x.

$$y = \beta_0 + \beta_1 \cdot x + \varepsilon$$

Table 7.5 Parallel distribution mark-ups Sweden

Calculation model		Consumer gains % of price difference	Wholesaler gains % of price difference	Parallel distribution mark-up
1	Average	33.4%	66.6%	35.2%
	Lowest	0.9%	3.0%	1.0%
	Highest	97.0%	99.1%	307.7%
2	Average	28.3%	71.7%	31.7%
	Lowest	0.9%	11.3%	1.4%
	Highest	88.7%	99.1%	237.0%
3	Average	36.3%	63.7%	28.3%
	Lowest	0.9%	3.1%	1.0%
	Highest	96.9%	99.1%	235.2%

Source: Own calculations, based on the national pricing authorities' data in Europe

The SPSS regression output shows that a 1% increase of the international price difference leads to a 0.75% increase of the parallel distribution mark-up. The regressions intercept is –0.05. We can therefore describe the relation between the international price difference and the parallel distribution mark up of a product which is brought into Sweden by the following function.

$$y = -0.05 + 0.75\,x + \varepsilon$$

Figure 7.3 The relationship between international price gap and parallel distribution mark-up in Sweden

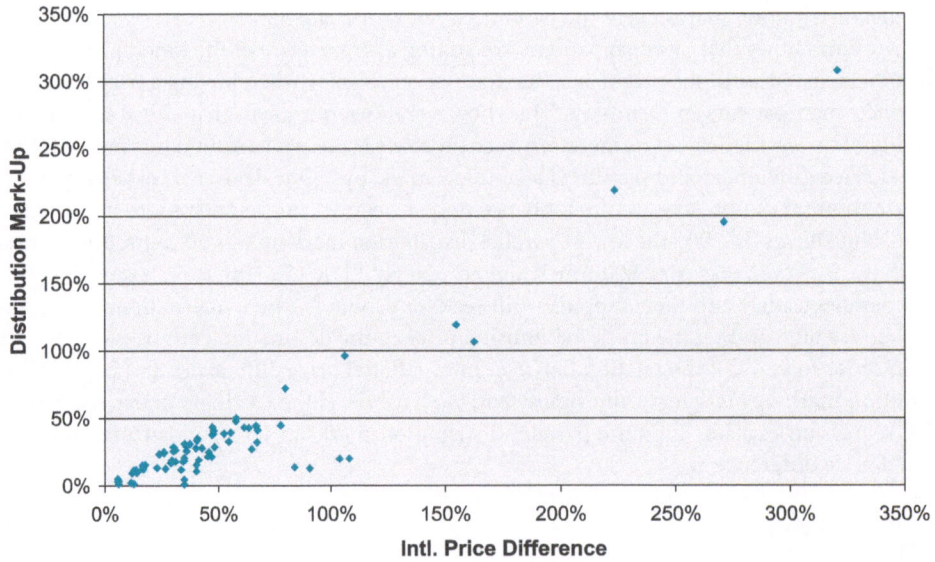

The statistical t-value for the slope (16.8) is larger than the critical t value for a significance level of 1% $t_{76;0.005} = 2.65$, meaning that we can, at a 1% significance level, say that there is a linear relationship between y and x. The statistical t value for the intercept (1.86) is larger than the critical t-value for a significance level of 10% $t_{76;0.05} = 1.67$. An analysis of the variance of the regression shows that we can, at a 1% level, reject the hypothesis that β_0 and $\beta_1 = 0$ since the critical F value $F_{0.01,1,76} = 7.01$ is smaller than the statistical F value (285). With 79.0% of the variation being explained by the regressor x we can say that the regression provides a sound explanation for the relation between international price differences and parallel distribution mark-ups. We observe that the slope of the Swedish regression is flatter than the regression for Denmark. This shows that competition among parallel traders is more intense in Sweden which makes it more difficult to attain a higher parallel distribution mark-up with larger international price differences. The findings described above are listed in Table 7.6.

Table 7.6 Regression analysis relation between distribution mark-ups and price differentials Sweden

Regression analysis					
Predictor	**Coef**	**StDev**	**T**	**P**	
Constant	−0.050		−1.863	0.066	
International price difference	0.753		16.88	0.0001	
		R-sq	0.790	**R-sq (adj.)**	0.787
Analysis of variance					
Source	**DF**	**SS**	**MS**	**F**	**P**
Regression	1	7.449	7.449	285	0.0001
Error	76	1.986	0.0261		
Total	77	9.435			

Source: Own calculations, based on the national pricing authorities' data in Europe

7.6   Price differentiation strategies by parallel traders

In the last chapters we have claimed that prices of parallel traded products are set by reference to the price of the locally sourced drug in the destination rather than the origin country. To prove that we need to show that the same parallel trader charges a different price for the same product in two different countries. There are a number of parallel traders who are active in all Scandinavian markets. By comparing prices charged by the two largest parallel traders in Sweden and Denmark[118] we are, therefore, able to tell if there is price discrimination going on or not. We use pricing information from the Danish Medicines Agency[119] and

---

118 June, 2005
119 http://www.laegemiddelstyrelsen.dk/1024/visLSArtikel.asp?artikelID=864, Accessed May, 2007

the Swedish Pharmaceutical Benefits Board[120]. Both government agencies provide monthly pricing information for all products at pharmacy purchasing and distribution prices. The average wholesaler mark-up in Sweden is 2.8% compared to 7.2% in Denmark. If a parallel trader charges the same to the wholesaler in Sweden and Denmark, the Danish pharmacy will have to pay 4.2% more than the pharmacy in Sweden.

If parallel traders did not practice international price discrimination the average difference between the wholesaler price for the same parallel traded product in Denmark and Sweden would, therefore, be in the neighbourhood of 4%. Table 7.7, however, shows that price differences between wholesaler prices in Sweden and Denmark are substantially higher. For parallel trader A, the average difference between the Swedish and the Danish wholesaler price is 12.0%. For parallel trader B, the average difference is 14.0%. The average difference for the locally sourced product is 8.1%.

Table 7.7 Differences of pharmaceutical prices between Sweden and Denmark

	Locally sourced	Parallel trader A	Parallel trader B
Average	8.1%	12.0%	14.0%
Highest	23.9%	35.0%	36.4%
Lowest	0.6%	1.8%	1.8%

Source: Own calculations, based on the national pricing authorities' data in Europe

These findings confirm our assumption that parallel traders are practicing price discrimination just as any other profit maximizing company would do. Furthermore it shows that price gaps of parallel traded products are larger than those of locally sourced drugs. This is because in 2005, Swedish prices were lower than those in Denmark and – at the same time – price gaps between locally sourced products and parallel traded products were higher in Sweden than in Denmark. Parallel traders will charge a higher price when selling their products to consumers in a market where price competition is weaker.

7.7   Outlook

Evidence presented in this chapter suggests that parallel distribution margins, as a percentage of the procurement price in the origin country, eased back between 1996 and 2005. Provided that this reduction cannot be explained by an increase in drug prices, engaging in parallel trade is now less profitable than in the 1990s. Competition has therefore induced parallel traders to operate more efficiently and to offer prices which are more attractive to the consumer.

Evidence in this chapter has also shown that for products imported into Scandinavia, there is a clear, significant and positive relation between the international price difference

---

120 http://www.lfn.se/LFNTemplates/ProductMedSearch____563.aspxm , Accessed May, 2007

for the locally sourced product and the parallel distribution mark-up. Moreover, it has shown that parallel traders practice international price discrimination too. This means that parallel distribution margins could ease back further, resulting in additional savings for the consumer.

Orifarm, Scandinavia's leading parallel trader reported a profit margin of 1.5% in 2005. While this may well be the consequence of wasteful spending and high managerial compensations, it also suggests that a part of the solution to obtain higher savings from parallel trade is to drive parallel *exporters'* margins down. Let us recall that parallel exporters are wholesalers, pharmacists and hospitals in the origin country. Evidence shows that because parallel importers' demand for pharmaceuticals exceeds available supplies, parallel *exporters* are able to sell to the highest bidder. Shortages in southern Europe would consequently drive prices of parallel traded products up. Whether and by how much parallel distribution margins will keep easing back in the future, will therefore depend on the future development of distribution and reimbursement structures in the destination country and the *availability of products in the origin countries of parallel trade*.

In this section we look at how recent legislative and regulatory trends on a community and at national level are expected to influence the future course of parallel trade in the European Union.

a) Recent court judgments

Between the 1970s and the 1990s, the pharmaceutical industry has virtually lost all litigations on parallel trade. These court rulings had allowed parallel traders to secure market access and prosper. With the Adalat ruling in 2004, however, tides have started turning in favour of the pharmaceutical industry. In this particular case, Bayer AG had adopted a quota system by which it reduced supplies of Adalat to its Spanish and French wholesalers. Bayer openly admitted that the aim of its quota system was to reduce exports to the UK. However, its standard terms and conditions did not prohibit exports. Parallel traders brought procedures against Bayer for breach of article 81 in the EC treaty. In 1996, the European Commission fined Bayer for having imposed an export ban as a part of its commercial relation with Spanish and French wholesalers. The case was brought to the European Court of Justice. ECJ decided that there was no evidence for an agreement between Bayer and the wholesalers in Spain and France. Indeed, wholesalers continued selling products even after Bayer had introduced its quota system. There was, therefore, no evidence for a meeting of minds between wholesalers and Bayer. In fact, the wholesalers sought to change their ordering policies in an effort to obtain extra supplies of Adalat that were intended to be exported[121]. The practice of limiting supplies to wholesalers was therefore legal.

A recent judgment by the Court of first instance of the ECJ has revoked the European Commission's decision to prevent GSK from pursuing a dual pricing strategy for pharmaceuticals in Spain[122]. GSK's dual strategy aims at ensuring that its medicines reach Spanish consumers rather than being diverted to more lucrative markets. The ECJ supports the Commission's view that the dual pricing system obstructed free trade. However, it finds that the Commission had failed to study the specific attributes of the pharmaceutical industry.

---

121 European Court of Justice (2004), Judgement of the Court in joined cases C-2/01 P and C-3/01 P
122 Court of First Instance of the ECJ (2006), Judgment of the court of first instance in case T-168/01

For instance, the Commission has failed to prove that dual pricing is not a necessity to finance research and development activities. In a communication that followed the GSK ruling, MSD informed its Spanish distributors that it will start charging what the company calls the European price. Distributors who can prove within 60 days that the drug has been sold in Spain, will receive a discount between the European and the Spanish price. Janssen-Cilag, Lilly and Sanofi-Aventis were also studying changes in the supply chain.

While parallel trade volumes are still growing – as the overall drug market is – the latest court rulings will have an influence on the availability of lower priced pharmaceuticals in typical supply countries of parallel trade. As long as the parallel importers' demand exceeds supplies, wholesalers in southern Europe can sell their products to the highest bidder, thus driving up prices for parallel traded drugs in northern Europe. Moreover, parallel traders are pushed into buying their supplies from other sources such as pharmacies and hospitals. Both hospitals and pharmacies charge higher prices than wholesalers. Product shortages in southern Europe are therefore a factor, which could impede further price reductions on parallel traded products in Europe.

b) Pricing and reimbursement reforms in Sweden and Denmark

The chapter on Sweden has shown that the introduction of the substitution and the reimbursement rule, combined with the implementation of an ordering system has led to an intensification of competition among parallel traders. The latest empirical evidence will raise politicians' awareness of what best practices are. We shall therefore expect governments to follow these best practices. As such reforms spread through Europe margins of parallel importers in Europe will keep easing back. A cross country comparison shows that the potential for further price reductions is highest in Norway and Germany and lowest in Sweden and the Netherlands.

c) Conclusions

Concerning the development of parallel distribution margins we can currently observe two trends. The first trend is that in the typical origin countries of parallel trade, pharmaceutical companies are now successfully setting up supply-control systems. Limiting the availability of products in southern Europe has the effect of containing parallel trade volumes. If supplies are scarce, wholesalers in Southern Europe can charge higher prices when selling a product to a parallel trader. Moreover, parallel traders will have to approach hospitals and pharmacists, a matter that drives procurement costs up. On top of this, pharmaceutical companies have started to use dual pricing as an instrument to make parallel trading unattractive. Overall, we shall therefore expect an increase of procurement costs for parallel traders.

At the same time, authorities in destination countries of parallel traders are implanting policies that have proven to be successful in inducing parallel traded competition. For instance, in some countries patients are now reimbursed to the level of the cheapest of all interchangeable products and pharmacies are requested to dispense that very same drug. Implementing such measures in other countries will add pressure on parallel distribution margins and drive savings from parallel trade up.

It is difficult to predict what the net effect of both trends will be. Pedersen's survey has shown that parallel exporters are responsible for 50–80% of the overall parallel distribution mark-up. Shortages of supplies in low price countries could, therefore, be a major hurdle to a price convergence between source and destination countries.

8

How should Switzerland proceed with its legislation on the exhaustion of patent rights?

8.1   Summary

Switzerland has adopted a policy of international exhaustion of trade marks and copyrights. Parallel imports of patented goods, however, are prohibited. Frustrated by high prices and drug expenditures, a number of payer and consumer organisations are seeking to adapt the patent law, so that parallel imports of patented goods would become legal.

In this last chapter we discuss how Switzerland could benefit from allowing parallel trade of pharmaceuticals. By using market shares and prices of parallel traded products observed in Europe as a reference, we develop a set of estimates for the impact that allowing parallel trade would have on Swiss consumers. Based on these findings, we develop policy proposals for Switzerland and Europe.

8.2   The Swiss healthcare system

8.2.1   Organization

Switzerland's healthcare system is financed by health insurance premiums, taxation and out of pocket payments. All permanent residents are obliged to purchase compulsory health insurance policies. Citizens are free to select a health insurance company of their choice and insurance companies are obliged to enrol any applicant for compulsory health insurance. Benefits included in the compulsory health insurance scheme are standardised for all insurance companies and laid down in the health insurance law (KVG). Health insurance companies compete with premiums and service quality (i.e. time until a service is reimbursed) rather than with benefits. To reduce the social impact of per capita premiums, cantons subsidise health insurance premiums through tax financed allocations[123].

Doctors in independent practices provide the majority of ambulatory care in Switzerland. Patients are free to choose their general practitioner and entitled to get a second opinion. Moreover, they have direct access to specialists. Ambulatory care is mainly financed

---

[123] European Observatory on Health Care Systems (2000): Health Systems in Transition: Switzerland, Page 28

by statutory health insurance, out of pocket payments and complementary insurance[124]. Health insurance companies are obliged to contract with all physicians who hold a license. Regulating bodies and health insurance companies have little influence on the number of physicians or on the type and amount of benefits which are provided by the primary care sector. Health insurance companies have, for instance, no means to refuse reimbursement to physicians who act inefficiently.

Concerning planning and funding, secondary care can be divided into two parts. The government has no planning authority on outpatient and short inpatient care (one night or less) and provides no funding for it. In contrast, inpatient hospital care (more than one night) is subject to state planning and receives government funding. Subsidies, however, are only paid to public hospitals while private hospitals are financed solely by health insurance companies and patients. Private hospitals which are listed in the canton's hospital list can be reimbursed for services under compulsory health insurance[125].

Prescription drugs are mainly financed by statutory insurance and co-payments when dispensed by a pharmacy or by a self dispensing physician. When dispensed by an inpatient clinic, the costs are equally split between the government that pays subsidies to the hospital and the health insurance/patient.

The result of a system with various payers, private providers and regulated benefits does not always provide incentives for treatment that is optimal for health or economically effective. The composition of the costs borne by health insurance companies does not reflect the effective contribution of different health providers to the health bill. This issue may lead to misguided lobbying by health insurers. For instance, they may pay less attention to addressing the inefficiencies in the secondary care sector than they would do if they had to pay the full cost that the hospital sector is generating.

Because of the hybrid structure of the health service sector – a combination of public and private ownership and funding – it takes more time to implement reforms than in a system which is either fully privatised or nationalised. Log-rolling among different healthcare providers is a common strategy to prevent reforms from happening, even if these may only affect the profitability of one healthcare provider. Physicians, for instance have – so far – successfully killed plans to abolish the obligation to contract – with the support of other providers of healthcare services and products. The inpatient sector is receiving support from allies in the healthcare industry in their struggle to delay the implementation of plans that would reduce the number of hospitals and hospital beds.

All in all, Switzerland is, therefore, a difficult environment for reforms that would induce price competition among and efficiency of healthcare providers. Switzerland lags behind Sweden in its implementation of policies which should induce patients and pharmacies to switch to the lowest priced of all interchangeable products and Swiss health insurance companies do not have the possibilities that US health insurance companies have to influence their members' behaviour.

---

124 European Observatory on Health Care Systems (2000): Health Systems in Transition: Switzerland
125 European Observatory on Health Care Systems (2000): Health Systems in Transition: Switzerland

8.2.2   Reimbursement of pharmaceuticals

The classification of pharmaceuticals in Switzerland has two dimensions. The first dimension explains whether a pharmaceutical is eligible for reimbursement or not. The second explains whether a pharmaceutical is available on prescription only or over the counter. While not all prescription drugs are reimbursed by the statutory health insurance, there are a number of over the counter drugs that are eligible for reimbursement. Pharmaceuticals which are eligible for reimbursement are published on the speciality list which is updated regularly.

Statutory health insurance requires patients to pay a fixed part of their annual health bill. The standard annual deductible for adults is CHF 230 p.a. Subscribers have the option of choosing a higher deductible in exchange for lower insurance premiums. The maximal deductible is CHF 1 500. Once patients have reached their annual deductible they are due to pay 10% of the price of all goods and services covered by the statutory health insurance. Maximal co-payments are capped at CHF 600 p.a. A patient who has opted for the lowest deductible will therefore endure out of pocket payments of no more than CHF 830 p.a.

For off-patent pharmaceuticals, a two tier co-payment scheme was introduced in 2006. According to this new rule, an increased co-payment of 20% is applicable to the *branded* drug if at least two thirds of all generic drugs are priced 30% or more below the branded pharmaceutical[126]. Co-payment for a generic drug, however, is always 10% no matter what the price difference between that generic and the branded product is.

The introduction of the two-tier co-payment system for off-patent drugs has increased demand for generic drugs at a patient level. To understand why, let us look at the example of the antidepressant Deroxat (14 tabs 20 mg) and its generic counterparts. Prices of and co-payment for the branded and all generic versions of Deroxat are listed in Table 8.1. On December 5th, 2006, the brand was priced at CHF 43.05. Out of the six generics available at that date, four were priced more than 30% below Deroxat. The most expensive generic was priced at CHF 34.05 while the cheapest one was available at CHF 20.90[127]. When buying the branded drug, patients would have to pay a price of CHF 8.60. For the most expensive generic a co-payment of CHF 3.40 is applicable. For the cheapest generic, the co-payment is CHF 2.10. By switching from the brand to the most expensive generic, patients can save CHF 5.20 or 60% of the co-payment, which is due for the brand. If the co-payment for the brand were still 10%, patients would only save 90 cents or 20%.

The development of generic sales and market shares from January 1st, 2006 shows that the introduction of the two-tier co-payment plan has affected the consumption behaviour of patients. In the year 2005 the share of generics on the Swiss market was at 8%[128]. In the first quarter of the year 2006, generic market shares were up to 12%, even though the multi-tier system had not even been implemented. The information alone that co-payments on branded products were about to increase, had the effect that patients would now ask their pharmacists for a generic more often. For the full year 2006, market share of generics was

---

126 http://www.sozialversicherungen.admin.ch/storage/documents/2408/2408_1_de.pdf, accessed 5.12.2006

127 http://www.bag.admin.ch/themen/krankenversicherung/00263/00264/00265/index.html?lang=de, accessed December 2006

128 Binder T. (2007), Pharmamarkt Schweiz 2006, IMS Health GmbH, Pages 7, 18

Table 8.1 Pricing and reimbursement for Deroxat and its generic competitors

Product	Marketing authorisation holder (Generic/Brand)	Price	Price advantage over brand	Co-payment (% of price)	Co-payment (CHF)
Deroxat	GlaxoSmithkline	43.05	0.0%	20%	8.60
Parexat	Streuli Pharma	34.05	20.9%	10%	3.40
Paroxetin-Mepha	Mepha	31.30	27.3%	10%	3.13
Parexat	Spirig Pharma	29.90	30.6%	10%	2.99
Paroxetin-Helvapharm	Helvapharm	26.75	37.9%	10%	2.68
Paroxetin-Sandoz	Sandoz	21.10	51.0%	10%	2.11
Paroxetin-Teva	Teva	20.90	51.5%	10%	2.09

Source: Federal Office of Public Health

11.6%[129]. After April 1st, an important share of patients believed that the 20% co-payment was applicable to all brands, irrespective of the price charged by the generic manufacturers. An individual generic manufacturer could, therefore, misuse the misperception of patients and set a price which is less than 30% below the price of the brand.

Because a co-payment of 10% is applicable to all generics, patients' incentive to switch from a random to the cheapest generic is generally weaker than his incentive to switch from the brand to a generic. In the case of Paroxetine, the co-pay for the most expensive generic, which is only 20.9% cheaper than the brand, is CHF 3.40. The co-pay for the cheapest generic, which is more than 50% cheaper than the brand, is CHF 2.00. By switching from the most expensive to the cheapest generic, the patient will save CHF 1.40. The health insurance company, however, would save CHF 11.80, if the patient decided to switch.

We find that the new two-tier co-payment system sets strong incentives to switch from a branded to a generic drug, whereas, incentives to switch from a random generic to the cheapest one are weaker. For this reason, we expect brand loyalty (i.e. a patients' inclination to buy a generic from a specific generic manufacturer) to be higher than in Sweden where patients pay the full price difference between the cheapest generic and the product they buy. Generic manufacturers are, therefore, expected to invest considerable sums in marketing to build a strong reputation and brand which will lower their ability to reduce prices.

8.2.3 The price setting process for pharmaceuticals

Prices of pharmaceuticals which are to be reimbursed by statutory health insurance have to be authorised by the ministry of health. The ministry uses two components to calculate the maximal price to be granted to a product.

---

129 Binder T. (2007), Pharmamarkt Schweiz 2006, IMS Health GmbH, Page 18

The first one looks at the average price charged in Denmark, Germany, the Netherlands and the United Kingdom. If prices for these countries are unavailable, or price differences among these reference markets to high, Swiss authorities may alternatively/additionally refer to the prices observed in France, Italy and Austria. The international price corresponds to the maximal price a pharmaceutical company may charge for any product which is eligible for reimbursement. The price is reviewed several times. The first review occurs two years after the product has received its marketing authorisation in Switzerland. Additional reviews occur the day that a product's patent expires and two years after.

The second component looks at how products used for comparable indications are priced. If the new product can prove to be more effective and/or safer than the old one, it may receive a higher price. If there is no evidence of any therapeutic progress, the product receives a comparable price.

8.2.4   The distribution chain of pharmaceuticals in Switzerland

a)   Wholesalers

Currently, there are four major and a number of minor wholesalers who are supplying pharmaceuticals and medicinal goods to retailers and hospitals in Switzerland. Galenica, Switzerland's leading wholesaler group owns and controls pharmacy chains and has developed into a full scale healthcare provider developing, manufacturing and marketing pharmaceuticals to the end consumer.

In the year 2002, a new pharmacy compensation system was introduced. Previously the calculation of pharmacy purchasing and distribution prices was based on the ex-factory price of a product. Both wholesaler and pharmacy margins were a function of the ex-factory price of a product. The new compensation system is now a combination of flexible wholesaler margins and flat pharmacy compensation payments (LOA). The so-called *"price to the public"* is the highest possible price that wholesalers can charge to pharmacies or self dispensing physicians. This price is calculated by adding a *distribution mark-up* to the ex-factory price. The *distribution mark-up* has two components: an 8–15% distribution mark-up on the ex-factory price (for products with an ex-factory price lower than CHF 1 800) and a staged compensation that increases with the ex-factory price. Wholesalers' margins are, therefore, still a positive function of the ex-factory price, meaning that they are interested in selling more expensive products. Wholesalers are allowed to charge any price, which is not higher than the official *"price to public"* to the pharmacist or the self dispensing physician. By charging the price to the public for the cheapest generic while charging a price lower than the price to the public for a more expensive generic, a wholesaler can induce pharmacists to dispense the more expensive generic. If, for example, the *distribution mark-up* for generic A is CHF 5 higher than the *distribution mark-up* for generic B, the wholesaler may consider sharing half of that amount with the pharmacist, so that the latter will opt for A. Table 8.2 illustrates how the *distribution mark-up* and the price to the public are calculated, given a specific ex-factory price. If the ex-factory price is CHF 20 for instance, the flexible distribution mark-up will be CHF 3 (0.15 · 20) and the staged compensation will be CHF 8. The official price to the public would consequently be CHF 30.

Table 8.2 Distribution mark ups for branded and generic prescription drugs in Switzerland (without LOA)

Price gap	Ex-factory price	Distribution mark-Up on ex-factory price	Fixed mark-Up
1	<5	12%–15%	4.00
2	5–10.99	12%–15%	8.00
3	11–14.99	12%–15%	12.00
4	15–879.99	12%–15%	16.00
5	880–1 799.99	8–10%	60.00
6	>1 800	No mark-up	240.00

Source: BASYS, Infras (2002), Auswirkungen staatlicher Eingriffe auf das Preisniveau im Bereich Humanarzneimittel

b) Pharmacists

Pharmacists have two sources of income. First, pharmacists can participate in the *distribution-mark-up* if wholesalers choose to set a price which is lower than the price to the public. Second, pharmacists receive financial compensations for dispensing pharmaceuticals (LOA). In 2006, the LOA compensation system had four different components.

- A pharmacist's allowance fixed at CHF 4.30 per prescription position
- A patient's allowance fixed at CHF 9.20 per customer and term
- A generic dispensation allowance, which amounts to 40% (no more than CHF 21.60) of the price difference between the generic and the brand. If the patient has a long-term prescription, the generic allowance is only paid once to the pharmacist, even if he continues dispensing the generic.
- An allowance for serving patients off hours

The generic dispensation allowance introduced in 2002, sets incentives to the pharmacists to dispense the lowest priced generic. Pharmacists are only allowed to cash the generic dispensation allowance once per prescription. If the patient holding a long term prescription receives generic "A" upon his first visit, and a lower priced generic "B" becomes available later on, the pharmacist will have no financial incentive to inform the patient about that product upon his second visit. We assume that the Swiss dispensation allowance is less powerful in inducing price competition among generics used on chronic conditions than the generic dispensation rule which is used in Sweden.

Moreover, offering compensation payments to pharmacists curtails savings from generic competition. Table 8.3 illustrates how the current pharmacy and wholesaler compensation system reduces the price advantage of a generic between the moment it crosses the factory gate, and the moment it crosses the pharmacy counter. The example shows that a generic which is 30% cheaper than the brand at ex-factory prices may, in the end, only be 10% cheaper to the consumer.

Table 8.3 Distribution mark-ups and end consumer

	Brand	Generic	Ratio Generic/Brand
Ex-factory price	15	10.7	0.7
Distribution mark up element A: regressive mark up (12%/15%)	2.3	1.3	0.6
Distribution mark up element B: progressive lump-sum payment (CHF)	16	12	0.8
Distribution mark up, total	18.3	13.3	0.7
Price to the public (official)	33.3	23.9	0.7
Generic Allowance (LOA element A)	0	3.6	
Pharmacy fee (LOA element B)	4.3	4.3	1.0
Patient fee (LOA element C)	9.2	9.2	1.0
End consumer price (effective)	46.8	41.2	0.9

Source: Own calculations

c)   **Self dispensing physicians**

In Switzerland, approximately 30% of all pharmaceuticals are directly dispensed by the physicians. Self dispensing physicians receive financial compensation for issuing a prescription but not for dispensing the product. Self-dispensing physicians will, therefore, charge the official *"price to the public"* to their patients. When dispensing a generic, self dispensing physicians are entitled to receive the same generic dispensation allowance as a pharmacist. Because a general practitioner has less space to store his pharmaceuticals than a pharmacy, he will have to be more selective with the products he chooses. We can, therefore, expect a self dispensing physician to only have the brand and perhaps one generic on site, which will generally be the one that the physician knows or trusts rather than the most cost effective. From the perspective of a generic manufacturer, it is, therefore, rational to concentrate its marketing activities on self dispensing physicians to elude price competition.

8.3   How well does Switzerland encourage parallel traded substitution and competition?

8.3.1   A simplified authorisation procedure

Parallel imports of patented pharmaceuticals are prohibited because the Federal Court of Justice has adopted a policy of national exhaustion of patent rights. Parallel imports of pharmaceuticals which are no longer under patent protection, however, are legal. The latter product group accounts for 43% of the Swiss drug market[130]. Statutory corporations which are

---

130   Binder T. (2007), Pharmamarkt Schweiz 2006, IMS Health GmbH, Page 18

interested in importing a lower priced pharmaceutical may apply for a simplified authorisation procedure. Applying for a parallel import license through a simplified procedure became possible in January 2002. Prior to that date, importing a pharmaceutical without the authorisation of the property right holder would have been prohibitively expensive because the applicant would have needed to go through the full authorisation process for new medicines. The simplified authorisation procedure, however, has reduced the costs involved in receiving a parallel marketing authorisation significantly. Simplified marketing authorisations are granted to applicants who can demonstrate that the parallel traded product fulfils the same safety and efficacy criteria as the locally sourced product[131]. In practice, a simplified marketing authorisation is granted if the product is sourced from a country where the medicine evaluation board applies safety and efficacy criteria which are comparable to those of Swissmedic. The countries and regions from where pharmaceuticals may be imported are: The European Union, The United States of America, Canada, Japan, Australia and New Zealand.

In order to allow Swissmedic to verify if the product that the parallel trader wishes to sell in Switzerland is equivalent to the domestic product, he is requested to submit data on the product including: the name of the product, the name of the product's property right holder, the manufacturer, information on the production process, active ingredients, concentration, expiry date, medicinal benefits and adverse reactions[132].

In addition, applicants are requested to submit a sample of the product which is intended to be marketed together with the translated patient information leaflet. All in all, requirements are therefore comparable to those in the European Union. Foreign pharmaceuticals which are equivalent to those on the domestic market, are eligible for parallel imports.

8.3.2 Directive to make all formulations of a product available

Parallel traders and generic manufacturers who intend to apply for a marketing authorisation for a specific product are requested to make all pack sizes, dosages and forms available to the patient. Because most products have various combinations of pack sizes and forms with low turnovers, it is often prohibitively expensive for a parallel trader to apply for a parallel import license. Moreover, not all pack sizes or dosage forms of a product with market authorisation in Switzerland, may necessarily be available abroad. No EU member country requires parallel traders or generic manufacturers to make all specifications of a product available. It is necessary to abolish the requirement to foster generic and parallel traded competition in the off-patent sector.

8.3.3 Lack of incentives to the middlemen and patients

The implementation of the generic dispensation allowance and the two-tier co-payment for off patent brands and their generic competitors, has triggered an impressive boost of generic sales and an impressive price reduction for off-patent pharmaceuticals. While patients now

---

131   Bundesgesetz über Arzneimittel und Medizinprodukte, HMG, Abs 14
132   http://www.swissmedic.ch/files/formulare/B3.1.125-d.doc, Accessed 17.04.2007

have incentives to buy generics and pharmacists have incentives to sell them, there is currently no law or legislation which would promote the procurement and distribution of lower priced parallel traded products.

Because pharmacists have neither directives nor financial incentives to dispense a lower priced parallel traded product, they will not exert pressure on wholesalers to have these products available. Wholesaler margins, moreover, are still a positive function of the ex-factory price. It is, therefore, in the wholesalers' interest to prevent pharmacists from ordering a parallel traded product. By charging the price to the public for all parallel traded products and setting a price which is lower than the price to public for the locally sourced brand, wholesalers can keep parallel traders out of the market. Evidence from Germany and Denmark has shown that wholesalers are likely to deny market access to parallel traded products if their margins are a function of ex-factory prices.

Moreover, same co-payment rules apply for parallel traded and locally sourced brands. If no generic version is available, the 10% co-payment is applicable for both the locally sourced and the parallel traded drug. If generics are available, the parallel trader has to offer a price, which is *"in the range of the prices"* charged by his generic competitors, in order to be eligible for a reduced co-payment of 10%. Because of co-payment rules for parallel traded products, patients are unlikely to actively ask pharmacists if a parallel traded product is available. Parallel traders are now in the same situation as generic manufacturers were in the 1990s.

We will, later in this chapter, present proposals for policy reforms which are a requirement for strengthening competition among different providers of interchangeable pharmaceuticals, may they be branded, generic, locally sourced or parallel traded. Before doing so, we will present empirical evidence on pricing patterns of generics in Switzerland.

8.4   Empirical evidence in Switzerland: the generic market

8.4.1   Summary

The generic market in Switzerland has experienced substantial changes since the beginning of the decade. Indeed, the generic market has been growing far ahead of the overall pharmaceutical market for seven consecutive years. The impressive boost of generic sales goes inline with the reform of the pharmacy compensation system in 2002 and the introduction of the two-tier co-payment system in 2006. In the first two quarters of the year 2006, market shares of generics were at 12.3% compared to 8% in 2005 and less than 3% in the year 2000. Moreover, the introduction of the two-tier co-payment system on April 1st, 2006 has induced price cuts for both branded and generic drugs (>500 price cuts). The rationale of generic manufacturers to reduce their prices is to push the branded drug from the 10 to the 20% co-payment bracket, so increasing patients' incentives to buy the generic rather than the brand. The rationale of the branded manufacturer is to move back to the 10% co-payment bracket in order to remain the patient's first choice.

The average price gap between the so called *"price to the public"* for branded and generic drugs was at 32.5% on September 1st 2006, compared to 60–80% in Denmark, Sweden and the United States. The generic dispensation allowance is not reflected in the *"price to pub-*

lic" meaning that effective price advantage of a generic product was still lower than 30% in September, 2006, despite the introduction of the two-tier co-payment system. It is particularly interesting to observe that generics seem to have settled 30% below the price level of branded drugs, which corresponds to the price gap required to push the branded product into a higher co-payment bracket. Savings from generic competition keep lagging behind their potential and there is still important room for improvement both concerning prices and volume shares of generics.

8.4.2   Generic sales

Generics had only played a minor role on the Swiss pharmaceutical market until the beginning of the decade. Indeed, market shares were lower than 3% less than six years ago and generics were mainly available for non-reimbursable, over the counter products. If generics had difficulties finding their way to the consumer, it is mainly because wholesalers, pharmacists and physicians had strong incentives to keep them out of the market and patients had only few incentives to ask for a cheaper prescription drug. The revision of the pharmacy compensation system in 2002, has allowed generic manufacturers to quickly increase their market shares from less than 3% in 2000 to 8% in 2005. While pharmacy margins had been a clear and positive function of the ex-factory price until the end of 2001, pharmacists had, for the first time, financial incentives to dispense a lower priced generic rather than the brand. It is only once the generic substitution allowance had been implemented that pharmacists started selling generic pharmaceuticals in larger quantities. Parallel to the introduction of the dispensation allowance, a law was passed, allowing physicians to practice generic prescription and pharmacists to substitute a generic for a brand without the physician's approval, provided that the GP issued the scrip using the non proprietary name. In 2006, generic sales increased by 46% and market shares are now 11.7%[133].

The recent experience with the generic market in Switzerland confirms that setting the right incentives to patients, pharmacists and wholesalers to switch to a cheaper product is an important precondition for generic manufacturers to gain market access.

8.4.3   Savings from generic substitution

According to IMS, the average generic was priced 40% below the locally sourced product in 2005. Savings from generic competition have totalled CHF 283 m, which corresponds to 5.5% of total drug expenditures. In September 2006, the average price difference between the generic formulation and the branded product had narrowed to 32.5% and by December 2006 the price difference was 28%[134]. This, however, does not imply that generic manufacturers would have increased their prices following the reform of the reimbursement law in April 2006. The reason why price differences between generics and branded drugs have narrowed is that the reform of the reimbursement law has induced manufacturers of branded

---

133   Binder T. (2007), Pharmamarkt Schweiz 2006, IMS Health GmbH, Page 18
134   Binder T. (2007), Pharmamarkt Schweiz 2006, IMS Health GmbH, Page 18

drugs to cut their prices by larger extents than generic manufacturers. Various manufacturers of branded pharmaceuticals were forced to cut their prices after suffering substantial losses in sales from January 1st 2006. The evidence shows that the reform of the reimbursement law has been successful in promoting generic substitution and in inducing manufacturers of branded products to reduce their prices. However, while the trend of the last couple of years may be impressive, adapting the current policy could increase the pressure on generic prices, thus generating further savings for the consumers.

First, as we have shown, patients still lack incentives to switch from a random generic to the cheapest one. The price cuts we have observed until now reflect the new competition between branded and generic manufacturers, a factor that explains why the price gap between generic drugs and branded products has narrowed. The previous chapters have shown that price cuts on branded drugs, which have gone off patent, can also be observed in Sweden or Denmark. The average price difference between the brand and the generic, however, is substantially higher in both Scandinavian countries. The difference between the Swiss and the Swedish reimbursement and dispensation law, is that Swedish patients and pharmacists have incentives/directives to *always* switch to the cheapest generic, no matter whether the patient has a one-time or a long-term prescription. For a generic manufacturer in Sweden, it is therefore more important to offer the best price than for the generic manufacturer in Switzerland.

Second, wholesaler mark-ups remain a positive function of the ex-factory price of a drug. The price charged by the wholesaler is somewhere between the ex-factory price and the so-called *"price to the public"*. Even under LOA, a certain share of a pharmacist's compensation remains, a function of the ex-factory price. Wholesalers are able to influence the pharmacists' purchasing behaviour by charging a price which is either closer to or further away from the price to the public.

Third, savings from generic competition are contained because pharmacists can keep 40% of the price difference between the generic and the branded product. The example in Table 8.3 has shown that there are cases where patients save as little as 10% on a generic which was priced 30% below the branded drug at the factory gate.

We conclude that despite the positive development on the generic market since the beginning of the decade, there is still room for further reforms on all levels of the supply chain, especially when it comes to reforms which could strengthen competition among manufacturers of interchangeable generics or parallel traded products. Proposals for these reforms are sketched hereafter.

8.5 Reforming the wholesaler/pharmacy compensation system and the reimbursement law

8.5.1 Decoupling distribution mark-ups from ex-factory prices

Table 8.2 shows that there is a clear and positive relation between the ex-factory price of a product and the distribution mark-up to the wholesaler. If generics have experienced such an impressive boost in the past years, it is due to the generic dispensation allowance. If parallel traders face difficulties gaining market access, it is because pharmacists have no financial incentives or obligations to dispense these products and wholesalers have incentives to sell the more expensive locally sourced brand to the pharmacist. In order to overcome this issue, distribution mark-ups have to be decoupled from ex-factory prices at all levels of the distribution chain.

8.5.2 Providing incentives to patients to switch to the cheapest, rather than to any generic (or parallel traded product)

Under the current system, a co-payment of 20% is applicable to the branded product, if at least two thirds of all generic products are priced 30% or more below the locally sourced drug. The co-payment for generics is fixed at 10%, irrespective of the price set by the individual manufacturer. It is, therefore, possible, for an individual generic manufacturer, to "free ride" on the prices set by their competitors.

When selling a product for which a generic is available, parallel traders need to price their products in the range of their generic competitors in order to avoid a 20% co-payment. This does not mean that the parallel trader will necessarily have to set the lowest price. We can, therefore, think of a situation where the patient who would otherwise have selected the cheapest generic, will now opt for the more expensive parallel traded brand. In this situation, the parallel traded product will have driven expenditures up, rather than down.

When selling a product for which no generic is available, the 10% co-payment is applicable for both products. The current reimbursement law does not provide any incentives to buy a lower priced, parallel traded product on top of saving 10% of the price difference between the locally sourced and the parallel traded drug. When a 10% co-payment was still applicable to all generics, demand for generics from a patient side was significantly lower than it is today.

In order to overcome the obstacles described above, we propose to limit reimbursement to the price of the cheapest of all interchangeable products, be it a generic, a locally sourced or a parallel traded brand. This measure would lead to an intensification of price competition and to a reduction of prices for generics and their locally sourced and parallel traded branded competitors. Physicians should have the option to object to generic substitution if doing so can be justified on medical grounds (e.g. generic or foreign brand does not work in individual patient because of different formulation).

8.5.3 Giving directives to pharmacists and wholesalers to dispense the cheapest, rather than any generic (or parallel traded product)

The generic dispensation allowance provides incentives to hand out the cheapest generic to the patient, whenever the patient uses a new prescription for the first time. The dispensation allowance may be effective in promoting generic substitution, however, in terms of inducing savings for the patients, it is highly inefficient. Furthermore, since there is no dispensation allowance for parallel traded drugs, pharmacists may simply refuse to order them, knowing that selling lower priced parallel traded products can result in lower distribution margins. Instead of randomly paying allowances for dispensing certain types of pharmaceuticals, the legislator should set directives to always dispense the lowest priced of all interchangeable products. Apart from easing market access for suppliers of lower priced pharmaceuticals, such a policy would induce competition and drive consumer savings up.

8.5.4 Summary

Our assessment of the Swiss system shows that because of inadequate incentives to patients and middlemen, sales of parallel imported non-patented pharmaceuticals are only picking up slowly. Moreover, compared to Sweden, the UK and the US, generic prices are high and utilisation rates low[135]. This should be kept in mind when assessing the potential savings from allowing parallel imports of patented pharmaceuticals. In the next subsections we present the legal options to the current policy of national exhaustion of patents. We assess the impact either path could have on the availability of parallel traded consumer goods and healthcare expenditures.

8.6 Assessing the legal options to the current policy on the exhaustion of intellectual property rights in Switzerland

8.6.1 The current situation in Switzerland and other industrialised countries

Exhaustion of property rights is a concept whereby the intellectual property owner loses the ability to control further sales of a product, following its first sale. Intellectual property rights may expire nationally, regionally or internationally. If a country has adopted a policy of international exhaustion of a specific property right, the intellectual property right holder cannot prevent a third party from buying his product abroad and importing it into that country. If a country has adopted a policy of regional exhaustion of a specific product, parallel imports from a selection of countries are legal. In either case, the intellectual property right holder may object to parallel imports, if the product in question has been put on the foreign market without his consent (e.g. the product was stolen). If a country has adopted a policy of national exhaustion of a specific property right, the property right holder can prevent parallel imports from anywhere.

Switzerland has adopted a policy of international exhaustion of trade marks and copyrights while patents expire nationally. It is therefore possible for Swiss distributors to source perfumes, clothing & footwear, cars, DVDs and electronics from anywhere in the world. Parallel imports of patented products, however, remain illegal. Overall, Switzerland's trade policy is more liberal than the trade policy of the US and the EU.

---

135 International Trade Administration, U.S. Department of Commerce (2004), Pharmaceutical Price, Controls in OECD Countries Implications for U.S. Consumers, Pricing, Research and Development, and Innovation, p. 23

The European Union has adopted a policy of regional exhaustion of intellectual property rights, making it impossible to bring consumer goods into the EU without prior authorisation of the intellectual property right holder.

In the United States of America, parallel imports of patented products are only permitted if the parallel trader has an import license for the United States. It is, therefore, fairly easy for a patent right holder to prevent parallel imports of patented products from happening. When it comes to products which are protected by trademarks, the property right holder can prevent parallel imports if the goods which are imported are not *identical* to those of the US trade mark owner. Solely by practicing marginal product differentiation (e.g. altering the country code of a DVD), the property right holder can prevent parallel imports from occurring.

Japan has – theoretically – adopted a policy of international exhaustion of property rights. In practice, however, patent holders can, by contractual agreements with their first buyers, prevent parallel imports. When it comes to the exhaustion of trade marks and copyrights, the law in Japan is unclear. However, evidence suggests that it is easier to prevent parallel imports of patented products than it is to stop parallel imports of products which are protected by copyrights and trademarks. Moreover, a very rigid authorisation policy of the medicine authorisation body in Japan makes parallel imports of medicines almost impossible.

Table 8.4 provides an overview of the policies on the exhaustion of property rights adopted in the leading economies of the world.

Table 8.4 Exhaustion policies of intellectual property rights in the world's leading economies

	Patents	Trade marks	Copy rights
The European Union	Community	Community	Community
The United States of America	National [a]	National [b]	National [c]
Australia	National	International	International
Canada	International [d]	International	International
Japan	National [e]	International	International
Switzerland	National	International	International

[a] Parallel imports are legal, provided the intellectual property right holder has given consent
[b] In theory, a policy of international exhaustion has been adopted. In practice, property right holders can prevent parallel trade from happening by practising marginal product differentiation.
[c] Supreme Court Ruling has levelled grounds for parallel importation
[d] While patents expire internationally, property rights holders may prevent parallel trade by the use of implied licenses
[e] Parallel imports are legal, if the property right holder has failed to make the adequate contractual precautions with his foreign clients

We conclude that all industrialised/emerging countries and territories, except Hong Kong and Argentina, have adopted a policy where patent right holders can prevent parallel imports from happening. Hong Kong's economy has – so far – been based on trade rather than innovation, which may explain the relaxed view of the country on the protection of patent rights. The claim that Switzerland has adopted a more restrictive exhaustion policy than other countries cannot be sustained. Indeed, Switzerland's most important trade partners, the European Union and the United States are both more restrictive towards parallel trade than Switzerland itself. We will, in the next subchapters present the legal options to Switzerland's current policy on the exhaustion of intellectual property rights. Furthermore we will present estimates on the savings resulting from implementing a policy of international or regional exhaustion.

8.6.2 The TRIPS agreement on the exhaustion of intellectual property rights

Switzerland has been a member of the World Trade Organization since its creation in 1995 and is bound to the legislation of the TRIPS and GATT agreements. The TRIPS agreement does not address the question of the exhaustion of intellectual property rights. Member countries may, therefore, implement whatever regulation on the exhaustion of intellectual property rights they choose. Member countries are also free to have different levels of exhaustion for each property right. However, according to Article 3 (National Treatment) WTO members may not grant nationals of a WTO member country a treatment that is less favourable than the one accorded to its own nationals. Article 4 (Most Favoured Treatment) quotes that with regard to the protection of intellectual property, any advantage, favour, privilege or immunity granted by a WTO member shall be granted immediately and unconditionally to the nationals of all other members. Switzerland is, therefore, not allowed to *unilaterally* implement a policy of regional exhaustion with EU/EEA countries.

The reason why EU/EEA has regional exhaustion is because the EC/EEA is considered to be a single market which is free to implement a policy of national (community exhaustion) or one of international exhaustion. Moreover, the EU itself is a WTO member. Expert interviews suggest that the EU is free to sign bilateral treaties on intellectual property rights, therefore stretching the common market for IP to other countries. Switzerland's attempt to reach such an agreement has already failed once in the 1980s when the European Commission decided not to open negotiations with Switzerland[136]. The reason for the Commission's disinterest is simple. European prices are lower than Swiss prices, meaning that European consumers could hardly benefit from such a treaty. In order to reach an agreement with the EU, Switzerland would have to offer something in return (e.g. further payments into the cohesion fund, concessions regarding tax competition and banking secrecy etc.). Moreover, it is unquestioned, that Sweden and Austria would insist on having all property rights included in a bilateral treaty with Switzerland. In order to reach an agreement with the EU, Switzerland would have to give up international exhaustion on trade marks and copyrights.

Concerning the adoption of a new exhaustion policy on patents, there are currently two alternatives to the status quo: joining the EU/EEA or implementing a policy of international exhaustion of patent rights. By joining the EU/EEA, Switzerland would automatically imple-

---

136 Parallelimporte und Patentrecht, Bericht des Bundesrates vom 8. Mai 2000 in Beantwortung der Anfrage der Kommission für Wirtschaft und Abgaben des Nationalrats (WAK) vom 24. Januar 2000

ment regional exhaustion of all intellectual property rights. A bilateral treaty on a regional exhaustion of property rights, under terms which are acceptable to Switzerland, would be difficult to implement. Given the current position of the Swiss population on an EU adhesion, implementing international exhaustion of patent rights is probably the only legally and politically feasible alternative to the current policy of national exhaustion of patent rights.

8.7   Modelling the economic impact of giving up international exhaustion on trade marks and copy rights

Should Switzerland join the EU/EEA or reach a bilateral agreement with the EU, the country would have to adopt community exhaustion for all intellectual property rights. Parallel traders would then no longer be able to import consumer goods from countries outside of the European Union. Parallel imported perfumes, cars, power utilities and (sports) fashion are helping Swiss consumers to save certain amounts of money. A majority of these products are sourced in the United States of America and South East Asia. Sweden and Austria both had international exhaustion on trade marks and copyrights before joining the EU in 1994. The *Silhouette* ruling, which was later confirmed in the Sebago[137] judgement, establishes that community exhaustion of intellectual property rights is binding for all EU member countries. Following these court judgments, Sweden adopted a policy of community exhaustion on July 1st, 2000, thus giving up access to lower priced parallel traded consumer goods from outside the EU/EEA.

8.7.1   The Swedish experience

In 1994, parallel imports of consumer goods from the US and Asia played an important role for consumers in the EU accession countries Austria and Sweden. Both countries pursued their policy of international exhaustion of trade marks and copyrights during the first years of their EU membership. However, in 1995 Silhouette brought procedures against Hartlauer for importing sunglasses from Bulgaria to Austria. Silhouette argued the fact that Austria had maintained its policy of international exhaustion of trade marks was irrelevant, because the EU had adopted community exhaustion. In 1998, the European Court of Justice ruled that in cases where the national exhaustion law was contradictory to Community law, the latter should prevail[138]. The ECJ ruling implied that all member countries should adopt a policy of regional exhaustion of property rights with the EU. In an attempt to demonstrate that preventing parallel imports from non EU-member countries was bad for consumers and the economy, the Swedish Competition Authority[139] commissioned a study. The study presented estimates on market shares of parallel traded products for different consumer goods, their origin and the savings resulting from parallel trade. It focused on product sectors that

---

137   The European Court of Justice (1999), Judgement of the court in Case C-173/98
138   The European Court of Justice (1996), Judgement of the court in Case C-355/96
139   Larsson, P (1999). Parallel Imports: A Swedish Study on Effects of the Silhouette Ruling

cover just over 43% of private consumption, according to the weighted average on which the 1998 price index had been based. The major sectors excluded from the study are housing, heating and household (33.6%), amusement and recreation (3.73%), travel and transportation (3.36%) and postal and telecommunication services (2.71%). These are sectors where, in all likelihood, there is no parallel trade. The importance of parallel trade of CDs and books has almost vanished due to internet trade. Based on the estimations of the Swedish Competition Authority, total value of parallel imported products accounted for 9 bn SEK in 1997, approximately 1% of total private consumption (SEK 925 bn). While parallel imports seem to have little importance in general, they account for a major share of total consumption of selected products such as automotive components (20%, two thirds originating from outside the EU), motorcycles (10% mostly from the US), clothing (10%, mostly from the US and South-East Asia) and footwear (5%, exclusively from the US and South-East Asia). The average parallel traded product was 15–30% cheaper than the locally sourced product and price gaps reached 60–70% for automotive components. Apart from the direct savings, parallel imported products have also been creating indirect savings for consumers. Parallel imported motorcycles, for instance, held a market share of 20–30% a few years before the survey. In 1997, mainly because of active competition and price adjustments, market shares were down at 10%. Price adjustments in Sweden were mainly a merit of parallel imports from the United States of America and would not have occurred under a policy of regional exhaustion of property rights with the European Union.

Parallel imports from countries that are not part of the EU/EEA accounted for 60% of total volume at retail prices in 1997. Parallel traders would therefore lose sales of SEK 5.5 bn which would force them to lay off 5 550 employees. Classical retailers would gain SEK 3.0 bn in sales and internet sales would go up by SEK 2.5 bn. Traditional retailers, whose profits would increase by SEK 100 m, would create 3 000 new jobs. Internet traders would also create new jobs – abroad. Imposing regional exhaustion of trademarks and copyrights would make the Swedish commerce lose SEK 2.5 bn in sales (EUR 289 m).

Moreover, banning parallel trade from non EU/EEA countries would inflict incremental expenses of SEK 350 m upon the unemployment fund and cause a reduction of 750 m SEK in tax revenues.

The Swedish experience suggests that preventing parallel imports from outside the EU has considerable undesired effects on the economy. According to the Swedish Competition Authority, the Swedish government would currently be falling short of 1.1 bn SEK (127 m EUR) in profits and Swedish retailers would be losing revenues of SEK 2.5 bn (289 m EUR) p.a. Total damage to the economy would amount to EUR 416 m, which is nine-fold of the savings from parallel imports of pharmaceuticals in 2003 (EUR 45 m).

8.7.2 Implications for Switzerland

The Silhouette ruling imposes a heavy burden on European consumers who are denied access to lower priced parallel imported consumer goods from outside the EU. By signing a bilateral treaty with the EU, Swiss consumers would no longer be able to buy parallel imported perfumes or cars from South East Asia and the United States of America. Prices for a selection of consumer goods would go up and consumer welfare down. Signing a bilateral treaty can only be justified, if savings from having access to parallel imported products from the EU that benefit from patents, exceed losses from no longer having access to parallel imported consumer goods that benefit from copyrights and trademarks from South East Asia and North America.

Concerning the importance of parallel imports of consumer goods into Switzerland and the savings resulting from it, there is no reliable data. A survey published by PLAUT-Economics in 2004 concludes that while unknown, savings are relatively low. The economic consultancy group finds that multiple regulations prevent parallel traders from sourcing products where prices are lowest[140]. Healthcare regulations, for instance, require foodstuff and cleaning agents to be labelled in the national languages[141]. It is, therefore, often impossible to import a branded product from a non-neighbouring country unless the box or the container in which the product is sold is re-labelled. Re-labelling a product is not only costly but may also entail a lawsuit for trademark infringement. Moreover, consumers may refuse to buy a product which has been manipulated. Parallel imports from overseas, as a consequence, is only common for products where re-labelling or repackaging is not necessary.

The majority of all products that do not have to be labelled in the national languages are imported from overseas. The majority of all parallel traded motor vehicles (5% market share), for instance, originate from the United States of America. Asia is an important supplier of parallel traded perfumes, shoes and clothes. The US plays an important role in supplying parallel traded power tools & home appliances, sports equipment and fashion. Unfortunately, no reliable numbers are available on parallel trade volumes or price advantages for most consumer goods. Certified figures are only available for crop protection products (3% market share) and foodstuff (5% market share) due to the obligation to declare such imports. The figures for crop protection products and foodstuff do not include private imports. Expert interviews conducted by PLAUT Economics suggest that overall volumes of and savings from all other parallel imported consumer goods are low. Immediate losses from no longer being able to buy parallel imported cars, fashion or perfumes from South East Asia or North America would, consequently, be negligible.

This, however, does not mean that gains from allowing parallel imports of patented pharmaceuticals would necessarily be higher than losses from banning parallel imports of consumer goods which are protected by trademarks and copyrights. First, products which are protected by copyrights and trademarks account for a larger share of private consumption than patented pharmaceuticals. Once all trade barriers have been eliminated, maximum savings potential from parallel imports of consumer goods is higher than maximum savings potential from parallel imports of pharmaceuticals. Second, market shares of parallel traded consumer goods are low because of regulatory entry hurdles. These entry hurdles impede imports of all products, not just those which are protected by trademarks and copyrights. Unless these market access barriers are removed, parallel traders will have difficulties importing patented pharmaceuticals too.

Legislators should, therefore, focus on tackling numerous regulations which are currently impeding market access for all types of products. Removing these market access barriers would result in savings for all products, not just those which are protected by property rights.

---

140 S. Vaterlaus (2004), Warum erodieren Parallelimporte die Preisinsel Schweiz nicht stärker? Ermittlung der Rolle der geistigen Schutzrechte anhand exploratorischer Expertengespräche

141 i.E. the official language of the canton, where the product is sold

a) Tolls
The Swiss Confederation levies import tolls for a variety of – mainly agricultural – goods. Import tolls are prohibitively high for certain products, meaning that foreign manufacturers are unable to market their products to Swiss consumers at competitive prices. Such tolls restrict market access for lower priced products from abroad, drive consumer prices up and delay structural reforms in Switzerland. An abolition of protective tolls is a requirement for making the overall economy more competitive and to drive prices of consumer goods down.

b) Declaration of the source of origin & tax discrimination
Parallel traders may not always be able to reveal the source of their products either because they are lacking the information or because they do not want to expose their supplier to sanctions by the property right holder. For a number of products, Switzerland applies different levels of taxation depending on where the product is imported from. Products which are imported from countries which have signed trade agreements with Switzerland, are generally subject to a lower taxation than imports from other countries. If a parallel trader is unable or unwilling to unveil the origin of his products, customs will impose the highest tax on that product. We can think of situations where the parallel trader ends up paying the standard import tax even though he has bought his products in a country that enjoys preferred taxation.

It would, nevertheless, be wrong to challenge the wholesalers' duty to declare the source of origin. Being able to trace a product back to the warehouse of the manufacturer is probably the most cost-effective way to ensure the authenticity and the safety of pharmaceuticals and to take the appropriate measures in the eventuality of a batch recall. Tax discrimination, however, should be eliminated unless it can be justified on competitive grounds. Tax discrimination is justified if foreign manufacturers receive (higher) subsidies (than domestic manufacturers) and in case there is evidence for dumping practices by the foreign manufacturer.

c) Authorisation procedure
For a variety of goods, wholesalers are requested to undergo an authorisation procedure before receiving the permission to import a product. A procedure that is known as the Cassis de Dijon Principle, allows manufacturers and wholesalers of products who have already received a marketing authorisation from an EU Member State to start selling that good in any other member state of the EU. Switzerland does not recognise market authorisations which have been granted by EU member states and often applies different technical standards. In order to release a product in Switzerland, manufacturers and wholesalers are therefore requested to undergo a full scale market authorisation and registration process during which they have to produce additional data. On top of that, they may also have to make adjustments' to their products so they can be released in Switzerland. The incremental costs of having a product adapted for and registered in Switzerland are borne by Swiss consumers. Complicated authorisation procedures are delaying and impeding direct and parallel imports of consumer goods and are responsible for a certain share of the mark-ups that Swiss consumers are paying compared to consumers in Europe. A harmonisation of authorisation procedures and technical standards and the mutual recognition of authorisations, could allow foreign competitors eased access to the Swiss market, accelerate structural reforms and have positive impacts on consumer and overall welfare.

We recommend that mutual recognition should be implemented in the context of a bilateral agreement with the EU. Europe is Switzerland's largest export market and domestic growth and prosperity depends on the ability of local firms to export their products to the EU. It would, politically, be unwise to allow European manufacturers eased access to Swiss markets without insisting that the EU grants the same right to Swiss manufacturers who intend to sell their products in Europe.

8.8   Modelling a policy move towards international exhaustion of patents

The economic impact of allowing parallel imports of patented products depends on a variety of factors such as total turnover generated by patented products, tradability of those products, the average price gaps between the potential source country and the destination market, the intensity of competition in the destination country, the relevance of regulatory entry hurdles and trade barriers and the level of cartelisation in the destination country.

On the last few pages we have shown that regulatory trade barriers are a major issue in Switzerland. The intensity of competition among different suppliers of substitutable goods or services is unsatisfactory and cartelisation a major annoyance. This must be taken into consideration when estimating the impact an authorisation of parallel imports could have on the economy.

In 2001, the Federal Council commissioned PLAUT-Economics a Swiss economic consultancy group, to present estimates on the consequences such a trade liberalisation would have on consumer prices and GDP. The study, which was published in 2002, presents estimates on the economic impact of switching from national to international exhaustion of patent rights. The follow-on study, which appeared in 2004, presents estimates of the economic impact of moving from national to regional exhaustion of patent rights. Unfortunately, the 2004 study does not include any forecast on the economic losses resulting from a move from international towards regional exhaustion of trademarks and copyrights. On the following pages we present the results of both surveys and assess the assumptions used on their comparability to what can be observed in the European Union.

8.8.1   Total turnover generated by patented products

In the year 2000, patented pharmaceuticals generated revenues of CHF 3.2 bn at retail prices. On-patent drugs represented 57.2% of the total drug market. Total revenue of patented consumer goods, however, can only be estimated. PLAUT economics identified five product groups where patent activity is high[142]. These product groups are clothing and shoes, furniture, power tools and home appliances, healthcare, transport and telecommunication and other goods and services.

---

142 Plaut & Frontier Economics, 2002, Erschöpfung von Eigentumsrechten: Auswirkungen eines Systemwechsels auf die Schweizerische Volkswirtschaft

Only a small fraction of all products that can be regarded as patent intensive have been granted a patent and only a proportion of these are still under patent protection. Transportation and communication, for instance, include fees for services such as ground/air transportation or telecommunication. These services are neither patentable nor tradable. While many automotive components are under patent protection, the assembled car is not patentable. A relaxation of the current policy would, therefore, merely affect the aftermarket components. PLAUT has narrowed the list of patent intensive product subgroups to fifteen, which together account for 32 bn CHF at retail and 18 bn CHF at wholesale prices. These products account for 12.9% of total private consumption. The list of patent intensive product groups includes chemicals, optical devices, HIFI-equipment, watches & jewellery as well as clothes and shoes. Patent intensity is particularly high for chemicals and optical devices but only moderate for fashion and electronic entertainment equipment. Furthermore, not all products that once received patent status are still under patent protection. Lacking reliable data on the total turnover generated by consumer goods which are currently protected by patents, PLAUT economics has, therefore, based its macroeconomic model on three different assumptions. The conservative scenario assumes that 20% (3.3 bn CHF) of all "patent intensive" products are still under patent, the traditional scenario 33% (5.5 bn) and the optimistic scenario 50% (8.3 bn CHF).

Table 8.5 Maximal arbitrage potential

	Pharmaceuticals	Consumer goods conservative	Consumer goods traditional	Consumer goods optimistic
Turnover patented products	1.9 bn	3.3 bn	5.5 bn	8.3 bn

Source: Plaut Economics, 2002, Erschöpfung von Eigentumsrechten, Auswirkungen eines Systemwechsels auf die schweizerische Volkswirtschaft

8.8.2 Economic impact of a policy move towards international exhaustion of patent rights according to PLAUT

According to PLAUT economics, a move from national towards international exhaustion of patent rights would trigger a 5.6 to 11.4% price reduction on patented products with a total trade volume of CHF 2.7 to 4.5 bn. Total savings would range from 153 m to 512 m CHF per annum. Because of reduced prices, private consumption would grow by CHF 11–131 m. Relative savings from parallel trade would be higher for pharmaceuticals than for classical consumer goods. Average prices of pharmaceuticals with total sales of CHF 1.6 to 2.3 bn would fall by 8–18.5%. Direct savings from pharmaceutical parallel trade would amount to CHF 130 m to 420 m. Health insurance companies and patients could, therefore, expect pharmaceutical expenditures to fall by 2.4–7.6%.

Table 8.6 Economic impact of a policy move towards international exhaustion of patents

	Pharmaceuticals		Consumption goods	
	Max	**Min**	**Max**	**Min**
Total revenue patent intensive goods at retail prices	5 500	5 500	33 000	33 000
Total revenue patent intensive goods at wholesaler prices	3 100	3 100	16 500	16 500
Total revenues of patented goods at wholesaler prices (maximal arbitrage potential)	1 850	1 850	5 500	3 000
% of maximal arbitrage potential that is exposed to PT	70%	50%	20%	10%
Total revenue of patented goods which are exposed to parallel traded competition (at wholesaler prices)	1 300	930	1 100	550
Average price difference World/CH at wholesaler prices	−40%	−40%	−30%	−30%
Average price spread between locally sourced and parallel traded products (at wholesaler prices)	−36%	−28%	−27%	−21%
Percentage of all products which are exposed to parallel traded that would be available at the reduced price	90%	50%	20%	10%
Average reduction of the price level at a wholesale level	−32.4%	−14.0%	−8.1%	−4.2%
Total revenue of all products which are available at the reduced price charged by the parallel trader (at retail prices)	2 280	1 630	2 200	1 100
Average reduction of the price at a retail level	−18.5%	−8.0%	−4.1%	−2.1%
Gross savings	420	130	90	23
Increase of consumption	41	0	90	11

Source: Own compilation based on Plaut Economics (2002), Pages 123, 131, 133, 134, 137

8.8.3   Assessing the assumptions used in the economic model used by PLAUT

PLAUT economics predicts savings of 2.4 to 7.6% on the overall drug bill, should Switzerland implement a policy of international exhaustion of patent rights. Savings from intra-community trade in the EU currently amount to 0.2–1.7% of total drug expenditures in the principal destination countries of the EU. It is likely that enabling parallel imports from throughout the world leads to higher savings than allowing parallel imports from the European Union only. The differences between PLAUT'S projections and current observations from Europe, however, seem to be too high to be attributed to this factor only. We shall therefore compare the assumptions made by PLAUT to our observations in Scandinavia and remaining EU.

a) Percentage of patented pharmaceuticals which are exposed to parallel trade

A look at Table 8.2 shows that pharmaceuticals, accounting for 50–70% of total Pharma revenues, would be exposed to parallel traded competition, if Switzerland adopted a policy of international exhaustion of patent rights. Observations from Europe suggest that products which are exposed to parallel trade, generally account for less than half of the drug market. The reason being that sales of products accounting for about half of domestic revenues are too low to allow a parallel trader to profitably compete with the licensed distributor. In Norway for instance, there were 2 555 pharmaceuticals registered in 2005. The 25 top selling products alone accounted for 29.4% of domestic sales. In Switzerland, there were 6 500 human medicines in 15 500 presentation forms available in 2005. The top 100 drugs accounted for approximately 50% of overall pharmaceutical sales, meaning that all other products generated average sales of CHF 0.3 m. The revenues that parallel traders could generate from importing these products would be too small to cover market entry, marketing and marginal costs of parallel distribution. In our estimate, the percentage of products which will be exposed to parallel trade ranges from 30 to 50% of the overall drug market.

b) Percentage of products exposed to parallel trade which are available at a reduced price

PLAUT predicts that between 50 and 90% (25–63% of the total market) of the products which are exposed to parallel trade would be available at the price of the parallel traded product. PLAUT expects the drug manufacturers to make their products available at the price charged by the parallel trader. However, the experience from Europe shows that this has, so far, not been the case. Observations from six major destination countries of parallel trade suggests that in Sweden, pharmaceutical companies have responded to parallel traded competition by reducing their own price, though to a level which is above the price set by the parallel trader. Observations in Germany, the Netherlands and Denmark suggest that pharmaceutical companies may seek to increase the price of a product which is exposed to parallel trade, in order to compensate for the resulting losses. The model in Chapter 6 has shown that pharmaceutical companies may prefer to accommodate parallel trade rather than deterring it. It has also shown that international reference pricing reduces a firm's incentives to deter parallel trade by modulating prices in source and destination countries of parallel trade.

During the past five years, a set of pricing reforms has driven Swiss pharmaceutical prices down. Sweden and Norway are already referencing their prices towards Switzerland. Other countries may decide to include the Swiss price in their calculation basket if the trend towards lower prices for prescription drugs in Switzerland persists. For these reasons and the ones presented in previous chapters, we do not believe that Swiss subsidiaries of pharmaceutical companies would react to parallel trade, by lowering the Swiss price to the level charged by the parallel trader. Taking market shares observed in the EU as reference, we believe that parallel traded products would account for 5–13% of total sales. 5–13% of domestic sales would be available at the price charged by the parallel trader[143].

Moreover, locally sourced products which are exposed to parallel trade could become available at a reduced price, which is higher than the price set by the parallel trader. We have made the assumption that 30–50% of the overall market would be exposed to parallel trade. With penetration rates of parallel traded products ranging from 5–15%, locally sourced products accounting for 25–35% of the overall market could possibly become available at a reduced price, which would be below the initial price of the locally sourced and above the price for the parallel traded product. Concerning the development of prices for locally sourced products, once parallel imports are permitted there are two possible scenarios. Either manufacturers will respond to the competition by reducing their prices or they won't. Our estimate is therefore that locally sourced products accounting for 0–35% of the overall market would become available at a reduced price which, however, is higher than the price charged by the parallel trader.

c) Percentage of the difference between the foreign and the domestic price which is retained by the parallel traders

PLAUT economics assume that parallel traders are unable to generate profits in the long run. Parallel traders would therefore be able to retain between 10 and 30% of the price gap between the supplier country and Switzerland. Latest estimates from the EU suggest that between 54 and 99% of the difference between the wholesaler price in the origin and the destination country of parallel trade is retained by the middlemen. Recent ECJ judgments, a shortage of supplies in the origin countries of parallel trade and the length of the parallel distribution chain, are responsible for parallel distribution costs being higher than what PLAUT originally expected.

d) Pharmaceuticals would be sourced from developing countries in case of a switch towards international exhaustion

PLAUT'S calculation of the average price gap between Switzerland and the World was based on a sample of 30 products. These products generated sales of CHF 470 m in 2000, representing 25% of the patented drug market. Wholesaler prices from eight countries[144] were taken from the IMS-Midas database. PLAUT assumes that each product would be sourced in the country where prices are lowest. 81% of all parallel imported products would originate from a developing country and only 19% from the European Union.

Swissmedic grants parallel import licenses through a simplified procedure if the product is sourced from Australia, Canada, EU, Japan, New Zealand and the US. These are countries where medicines evaluation bodies apply product safety and efficacy standards which are comparable to these applied by Swissmedic. However, Swissmedic does not grant parallel import licenses if the parallel trader intends to source his product in an emerging or developing country. The list of countries that are not eligible for a parallel import license through a simplified procedure includes Brazil, Russia, India, China, Mexico and South Africa. Because standards used by medicine control agencies in these countries are inferior to the ones

---

143   20% of all pharmacy sales are parallel traded
144   South Africa, Brazil, India, Greece, Spain, Hong Kong, Poland, Bulgaria

used by Swissmedic and because developing countries have severe issues with counterfeit drugs[145], Swiss regulators seem to believe that it would not be possible to ensure the protection of public health if parallel imports from developing countries through a simplified authorisation procedure became possible. We assume that the list of countries which are eligible for a simplified marketing authorisation would not be modified after a policy move towards international exhaustion. Experience shows that the possibility to apply for a simplified marketing authorisation is a pre-condition for parallel trade to happen. Technically, parallel traders would then be able to source products from the industrialised countries mentioned above.

Price levels in Japan and the United States of America (list prices) are higher than in Switzerland. The two largest drug markets in the world are therefore not suitable for parallel imports into Switzerland. Drug prices in Canada are comparable to the EU and average prices in Australia and New Zealand comparable to prices in Southern Europe. Costs of sourcing a product from Australia, Canada or New Zealand, however, would be higher than costs of sourcing a product from Spain or Italy because of longer transportation routes. Moreover, established parallel traders have no business relations with wholesalers in Oceania and Canada. Based on these reflections we believe that the bulk of all parallel imports would emerge from European Union Member States, should Switzerland impose a policy of international exhaustion of patent rights.

In 2004, PLAUT published a follow-up survey which estimated savings from parallel trade of medicines, should Switzerland implement a policy of regional exhaustion of patents with the EU. In Chapter 8.9 we present PLAUT's estimates on the economic impact of implementing regional exhaustion of patent rights. These estimates can also serve as proxy of the economic impact of implementing international exhaustion.

8.9 Modelling a policy move towards regional exhaustion of patents

In order to ensure comparability with the previous study PLAUT Economics uses revenue figures and pricing information that was utilised in the 2002 report. Table 8.7 gives an overview of how an eventual relaxation of the patent law would affect drug prices and drug expenditures in Switzerland.

According to PLAUT, a liberalisation of the current exhaustion policy for patented products would therefore induce savings of CHF 57.7 m to 222.7 m or CHF 8 to 30 per capita and year. This implies that implementing regional exhaustion of patent rights with the EU would reduce drug expenditures by 1.1 to 4.1%. The lower estimate made by PLAUT is in the range of what can currently be observed in Europe. In 2002, savings from parallel traded drugs represented 1.7% of overall drug expenditures in the Netherlands[146] and Swe-

---

145 http://www.who.int/mediacentre/factsheets/fs275/en/ , accessed on 27.01.2006

146 Kanavos P. and Costa-Font J (2005), Pharmaceutical parallel trade in Europe: stakeholder and competition effects, Economic Policy October 2005, p 778

Table 8.7 Economic impact of a policy move towards regional exhaustion of patents

	PI of medicines given regional exhaustion	
	Max	Min
Total pharmaceutical market at retail prices	5 456	5 456
Total pharmaceutical market at wholesaler prices	3 121	3 121
Total patented market at wholesaler prices	1 854	1 854
Price difference EU/CH at wholesaler prices	−25%	−25%
Origin of patented products		
Domestic production (31%)	575	575
Foreign production (69%, EU 40%, non EU 29%)	1 279	1 279
Total volume affected by policy change[a]	1 586	1 318
Total arbitrage potential[b]	**1 110**	**659**
Price difference between locally sourced and parallel traded products[c]	22.5%	17.5%
Average price reduction due to PI at wholesale prices [d]	**−20.5%**	**−8.75%**
Average savings due to PI at wholesaler prices	**228.6 m**	**58.6 m**
Savings/total market at wholesale prices	**7.3%**	**1.8%**
Average price reduction due to PI at pharmacy prices[e]	**−11.58%**	**5.01%**
Average savings due to PI at pharmacy prices	**222.7 m**	**57.7 m**
Savings/total market at pharmacy prices	**−4.1%**	**−1.1%**

[a] Assuming that 50%/0% all products manufactured outside the EU may still be imported (HI/LO)
[b] Assuming that 70%/50% off total arbitrage potential may be sourced regardless of remaining trade barriers
[c] Assuming that 10/30% of the international price difference is need to cover the international price differences
[d] Assuming that 90/50% of all products become available at the reduced price
[e] Assuming that 90/50% of all products become available at the reduced price
Source: Vaterlaus, S (2004): Auswirkungen eines Wechsels zur regionalen Erschöpfung im Patentrecht, PLAUT

den, 1.5% in the United Kingdom[147], 0.9% in Denmark, 0.6% in Germany[148] and 0.2% in Norway. Overall, parallel traded pharmaceuticals generated sales of EUR 4.2 bn and savings of EUR 455 m, which is 1.0% of total drug expenditures in these six countries. These results are summarised in Table 8.4.

---

147 Kanavos P. and Costa-Font J (2005), Pharmaceutical parallel trade in Europe: stakeholder and competition effects, Economic Policy October 2005, p 778

148 Kanavos P. and Costa-Font J (2005), Pharmaceutical parallel trade in Europe: stakeholder and competition effects, Economic Policy October 2005, p 778

Table 8.8 Savings from parallel trade in Europe (2002), in m EUR at pharmacy purchasing prices

	Sales PI	Market share PI	Sales total market	Av price advantage	Savings PI	Savings PI in % of total drug market
DE	1 332	7.10%	18 761	6.70%	95.7	0.5%
DK	178	9.40%	1 894	8.80%	17.2	0.9%
NL	267	9.00%	2 967	15.80%	50.1	1.7%
NO	78	6.30%	1 238	3%	2.4	0.2%
SE	228	9.10%	2 505	15.70%	42.5	1.7%
UK	2 154	13.10%	16 443	10.3%	246.6	1.5%
Total	4 237	9.67%	43 807	9.7%	455	1.0%

Source: Own compilation based on Kanavos & Costa-Font, EFPIA, DLI, LS and Farmastat

The chapters on Sweden, Norway and Denmark have shown that savings from parallel trade are a function of market size, the number of market actors and the incentives given to physicians, pharmacists and patients to act cost responsibly. Table 8.4 shows that while savings from parallel trade are sizeable in Sweden and the Netherlands, savings are low in Norway and – in relative terms – in Germany.

In Sweden, pharmacies are legally obligated to always dispense the lowest priced of all interchangeable drugs. Interchangeable drugs, in Sweden, are products with same active ingredient, dosage, form and pack size as the locally sourced brand. Patients are reimbursed up to the price of the cheapest product available and co-payment is high. In the Netherlands, pharmacists are reimbursed up to the price of the cheapest interchangeable product. Pharmacists who dispense another than the cheapest of all interchangeable products, pay the difference out of their own pocket.

In Germany, wholesalers and pharmacy margins are a positive function of the ex-factory price of a pharmaceutical. Market shares of parallel traded pharmaceuticals and the price difference between locally sourced and parallel traded products are governed by the authorities. In Norway, wholesaler chains are able to retain price reductions offered by parallel traders and use them for their own purpose. Norwegian patients have only few incentives to switch from a locally sourced brand to a lower priced parallel traded product.

High price advantages of parallel traded pharmaceuticals in Sweden and the Netherlands are the reward of setting appropriate incentives on all levels of the supply chain. Low price advantages and market shares in Germany and Norway are the consequence of an inappropriate policy.

Our assessment on the current policy set up in Switzerland shows that wholesalers have financial incentives to keep parallel traders out of the market. Patients can only save 10% of the price difference between the locally sourced and the parallel traded drug when buying the latter. Physicians are either indifferent or inclined towards dispensing the locally sourced product. Moreover, market access for parallel traders is hampered by a requirement to make all formulations of a product available. The current policy set up does not support parallel traded substitution or competition. It is, therefore, necessary to model the economic impact of a policy move towards international or regional exhaustion of patent rights using minimal and maximal savings observed in the EU as benchmark.

Table 8.9 illustrates what Switzerland could expect in terms of savings if a policy of regional or international exhaustion of patents was implemented. A switch from national towards international or regional exhaustion of patents would affect *patented* pharmaceuticals only. For this reason, we look at the market for patented pharmaceuticals only. In 2000, patented pharmaceuticals generated sales of CHF 1 854 m at wholesaler prices.

From all patented pharmaceuticals which were sold in 2000, those manufactured in Switzerland held a market share of 31%, those manufactured in the EU 40% and those manufactured in the rest of the world 29%. Not all products which have a marketing authorisation in Switzerland are also available in Australia, EU/EEA, North America, Japan or New Zealand. Moreover, it is possible that market authorisation will only be granted to parallel traders who make all formulations of a product available. This would have considerable implications on the business potential of parallel traders in Switzerland. Let us therefore assume that 70–98%, off all products with a marketing authorisation in Switzerland could be obtained from a wholesaler abroad and imported into the country after assessment by Swissmedic. Total revenue of all patented products that would be eligible for parallel trade would therefore range from CHF 1 298 to CHF 1 817 as seen in Table 8.5.

Table 8.8 shows that market shares of parallel imported pharmaceuticals on the overall market, range from 6–13% in the six principal destination markets of parallel trade. Using Europe as a reference, we can therefore assume that 6–13% of all pharmaceuticals sold in Switzerland would be parallel imported drugs.

The market shares observed in Europe refer to the overall drug market. Because parallel import penetration is higher in the patented, than in the off-patent market we need to adjust the figures which are observed in Europe, so that they can be used for our model. Let us, therefore, think of a scenario, where parallel import penetration is 25% higher among patented than among off patented pharmaceuticals and of a second scenario where parallel import penetration is three times higher. Knowing that patented products account for 57% of the pharmaceutical market and market shares of parallel traded products would range from 6–13%. We derive the following formulas to calculate the penetration rate γ of parallel imported products on all patented products.

Conservative: $(0.8 \cdot y) \cdot 0.43 + y \cdot 0.57 = 0.06 \quad \longleftrightarrow \quad y = 0.07$

High: $(0.3 \cdot y) \cdot 0.43 + y \cdot 0.57 = 0.13 \quad \longleftrightarrow \quad y = 0.18$

The share of parallel imported pharmaceuticals on the market for *patented* pharmaceuticals would, therefore, range from 7 to 18%. Sales of parallel traded and patented pharmaceuticals, as a consequence, would amount to CHF 148–332 m at prices of locally sourced drugs.

Recent empirical evidence shows that price gaps between the locally sourced and the parallel traded product range from 2–16% in the six major destination countries of parallel trade. Swiss prices are comparable to prices in the major destination countries of parallel trade. Moreover, most products imported into Switzerland would emerge from the EU. We may therefore assume that the average parallel traded product in Switzerland would be priced 2–16% below the locally sourced product.

By multiplying the lowest expected price gap (2%) with the lowest expected turnover of parallel traded products, which at prices of locally sourced products is CHF 121 m, we find that direct savings from parallel trade at wholesaler prices would, in the worst case, be CHF 2.4 m. By multiplying the highest expected price gap with the highest expected turnover we find that direct savings from parallel trade would, in the best case, be CHF 53 m. As a percentage of total expenditures on pharmaceuticals, Switzerland could therefore expect direct savings of 0.1–1.7%.

On top of the direct savings, parallel imports of pharmaceuticals could also induce indirect savings due to price reductions granted by the Swiss subsidiaries of the pharmaceutical companies. Ganslandt and Maskus[149] find that competition from parallel trade would have contained price growth of locally sourced pharmaceuticals by 1.2% between January 1996 and December 1997. In Chapter 3 we found the average time-span between market entry and market exit for a parallel traded product in Denmark is three years. The average parallel traded product has therefore been on the market for one and a half years. When using findings by Ganslandt and Maskus as a reference, we find that the price of a locally sourced product, which is exposed to parallel trade, is approximately 1% lower than it would be without being exposed to this competition. Empirical evidence from other countries suggests that pharmaceutical companies may not necessarily respond to parallel traded competition by reducing their prices. Let us therefore assume that parallel imports will trigger a price reduction of 0–1% on all locally sourced products which are exposed to parallel trade. Table 8.5 shows that locally sourced patented drugs which are generating sales of up to CHF 1.485 m could be exposed to parallel traded competition. Assuming that prices of these products ease back by 1%, indirect savings would amount to CHF 14.9 m. Total savings at wholesaler prices from parallel trade would consequently range from CHF 2.4–69 m. PLAUT shows that savings at wholesaler prices are comparable to savings at retail prices because of the structure of the pharmacy compensation system. Savings per head and annum would, therefore, be in the range between CHF 0.30 and CHF 9.50. These findings are summarised in Table 8.9.

We reckon that the spread between the optimistic and the pessimistic estimation is high, but so are the differences in terms of savings between different EU countries. The last chapters have shown that incentives to the patients to buy the lowest priced of all interchangeable products, directives to pharmacists to dispense that very same product, the absence of financial incentives to *any* of the middlemen to dispense higher priced products and the prohibition of discounts are essential preconditions for effective competition on the market for parallel traded pharmaceuticals. In Switzerland, none of these conditions is met. Even though patients may –meanwhile – have incentives to buy lower priced generics this is not the case for (off-patent) parallel traded products. Should Switzerland allow parallel imports under the current framework, savings would probably be low. By implementing structural reforms such as the ones presented in Chapter 8.5, Switzerland could probably attain sizeable savings from implementing regional or international exhaustion of patents. Theses savings would probably be in region of CHF 70 m p.a., representing 2% of pharmaceutical expenditures.

---

149 M. Ganslandt, K.E. Maskus (2004), J. of Health Economics 23 (2004) 1035–1057, p.1049

Table 8.9 Revised projections for a policy move towards regional exhaustion of patents

All values in m CHF at wholesaler prices (unless specified otherwise)	MIN	MAX
Total revenue patented pharmaceuticals	1 854	1 854
Percentage of all patented products eligible for parallel imports	70%	98%
Total market value of patented pharmaceuticals eligible for parallel imports	1 298	1 817
Sales of parallel traded products as a share of total sales of patented pharmaceuticals	7%	18%
Revenue of patented parallel traded pharmaceuticals at prices of locally sourced drugs	148	332
Average price advantage of parallel imported products	2%	16%
Direct savings from patented & parallel traded products	2	54
Direct savings from patented & parallel traded products as a share of overall drug expenditures	0.1%	1.7%
Revenue of locally sourced & patented products which are exposed to parallel trade	1 150	1 485
Price reduction on locally sourced products after market entry of parallel trade	0%	1%
Indirect savings from parallel trade	0	15
Total savings from parallel trade	2	69
Total savings from parallel trade of patented products as a share of overall drug expenditures	0.1%	2.2%

Source: Own projections

8.10   Conclusions and policy proposals for Switzerland

Evidence from Scandinavia shows that savings from parallel trade vary considerably depending on the regulatory and the market environment in a country. Savings form parallel trade are sizeable in Sweden, moderate in Denmark and low in Norway. A policy assessment shows that the market environment in Switzerland is not supportive to parallel traded substitution and competition. Currently, neither pharmacies nor wholesalers have any obligations or incentives to dispense lower priced parallel imported brands. The generic dispensation allowance which has helped to boost generic sales is questionable because an important share of the price reduction granted by the manufacturer ends up in the pharmacists' rather than in the patients' pocket. Moreover, we find that an important share of the savings attained during the last two years results from originators, rather than generic manufacturers lowering their prices[150]. A report by the International Trade Commission of the U.S. De-

---

150   Binder T. (2007), Pharmamarkt Schweiz 2006, IMS Health GmbH, Pages 7, 18

partment of Commerce, shows that generic prices in Switzerland are 50–70% higher than in the United States of America[151]. IMS health reports that generic prices have only eased back moderately since January 2005, meaning that Swiss prices of generics keep exceeding US prices by a long shot. Evidence shows that Switzerland lags far behind Sweden, the United Kingdom and the United States when it comes to generic competition. Low market shares and excessive prices for generics are not a coincidence but the consequence of a misguided health policy and a series of patchwork reforms.

We recommend that Switzerland should, in a first step, implement the reforms described in Chapter 8.5. By doing so, Switzerland could attain substantial savings by bringing generic utilisation rates up, and generic prices down to US or Swedish levels. In a second stage, Switzerland should, under an improved competitive situation, re-evaluate the option of a relaxation of the current patent law. This evaluation should take account of both short and long term impacts that such a decision may have.

---

[151] International Trade Administration, U.S. Department of Commerce (2004), Pharmaceutical Price, Controls in OECD Countries Implications for U.S. Consumers, Pricing, Research and Development, and Innovation, p. 23

9
References

9.1 Bibliography

Addor, F (2004): "Parallelimporte patentierter Waren: Eine unendliche Geschichte?, Speaking notes, press seminar "Parallelimporte Patentgeschützter Medikamente", Berne, June 29th, 2004

Binder T. (2007): Pharmamarkt Schweiz 2006, IMS Health GmbH, Hergiswil http://www.ihaims.ch/Uploads/N274.pdf

Bouvy. F (2003): Overview of pricing and reimbursement measures taken since January 1993, European Federation of Pharmaceutical Industry Associations (EFPIA), Brussels

Bouvy. F (2003): Reference Price Systems, an overview, Federation of Pharmaceutical Industry Associations (EFPIA), Brussels

Bundesamt für Gesundheit (2001): Die Obligatorische Krankenversicherung kurz erklärt, Berne

Bundesministerium für Justiz: Sozialgesetzbuch – Fünftes Buch (V) – Gesetzliche Krankenversicherung (Artikel 1 des Gesetzes v. 20. Dezember 1988, BGBl. I S. 2477), http://bundesrecht.juris.de/sgb_5/, accessed on 20.02.2006

Cambridge Pharma Consulting (2002): Delays in Market Access, Cambridge, UK

College Tarieven Gezondheidszorg: Tariefbeschikking, www.ctg-zaio.nl, accessed on 13.02.2006

Danzon, P. (1997): Pharmaceutical Price Regulation, National Policies versus Global Interests, Washington

Danzon, P. (2001): Reference Pricing Theory and Evidence, Wharton School, University of Pennsylvania, Philadelphia

Department of Health (2006): 2005 Consultation Document Arrangements for the Provision of Dressings, Incontinence Appliances, Stoma Appliances, Chemical Reagents and Other Appliances to Primary and Secondary Care, London

DiMasi. J, (2002): Price trends for prescription pharmaceuticals: 1995–1999, a background report for the department of health and human services, http://aspe.hhs.gov/health/reports/Drug-papers/dimassi/dimasi-final.htm, accessed on 13.02.2006

DiMasi, J. (2004): The economics of follow-on drug research and development, Pharmacoeconomics 2004; 22 Suppl. 2: 1–14

DiMasi, J et al. (2003): The price of innovation: New estimates of drug developing costs, J. of Health Economics, 22 (2003) 151–185

Eidgenössisches Volkswirtschaftsdepartement (2000): Parallelimporte und Patentrecht. Bericht des Bundesrates vom 8. Mai 2002 in Beantwortung der Anfrage der Kommission für Wirtschaft und Aufgaben des Nationalrates (WAK) vom 24. Januar 2000

European Commission (1982): European Commission Communication AB1 Nr. C 115, 06.05.1982

European Court of Justice (1974): Judgement of the Court In Case 15/74, between Centrafarm BV et Adriaan de Peijper v Sterling Drug Inc.

European Court of Justice (1998): Judgement of the Court In Case C-355/96, between Silhouette International Schmied GmbH & Co. KG

European Court of Justice (1999): Judgement of the Court in Case C-173/98, between Sebago Inc. and Ancienne Maison Dubois et Fils SA and GB-Unic SA

European Court of Justice (2001): Judgement of the Court in Case 15/01, between Paranova Läkemedel et al. vs. Läkemedelsverket

European Court of Justice (2002): Opinion of Advocate General Léger in Case C-438/02, between Åklagaren v Krister Hanner

European Court of Justice (2004): Judgement of the Court in joined Cases C-2/01 P and C-3/01, between Bundesverband der Arzneimittel-Importeure eV et al. and Bayer AG et al.

European Court of Justice (2006): Judgment of the Court of First Instance in Case T-168/01, between GlaxoSmithKline Services Unlimited and the Commission of European Communities et al.

European Federation of Pharmaceutical Industries Association, EFPIA (2006): The Pharmaceutical Industry in Figures, 2006 Edition, Brussels

Frank R.G., Salkever D.S. (1997): Generic Entry and the Pricing of Pharmaceuticals, J. of Econ & Management Strategy, Spring, pp.75–90

Gansladt M, Maskus K (2001): Parallel Imports of Pharmaceuticals in the European Union, Working Paper No 546, 2001, The Research Institute of Industrial Economics, Stockholm

Ganslandt M., Maskus K.E. (2004): Parallel Imports of Pharmaceuticals in the European Union, J. of Health Economics 23 (2004) 1035–1057

Glenngård A. et al. (2005): Health Systems in Transition: Sweden, Vol. 7 No. 4, Page 48, European Observatory on Health Systems and Policies, Copenhagen

Glynn D. et al. (1997): Survey of parallel trade, National Economic Research Associates NERA, London

Haigh, J. (2003): Parallel Trade in Europe, Strategies for Global Corporations, IMS Health, London

Huskamp, A et al. (2003): The Effect of Incentive-Based Formularies on Prescription-Drug Utilisation and Spending, N Engl. J Med 2003;349:2224–32.

Roth Johnsen J. (2006): Health Systems in Transition: Norway, Vol. 8 No. 1 2006, The European Observatory on Health Systems and Policies, Copenhagen, Denmark

IMS Consulting (2003): A comparison of pharmaceutical pricing in Switzerland with selected reference countries, London

Infras/Basys (2002): Auswirkungen staatlicher Eingriffe auf das Preisniveau im Bereich Humanarzneimittel, Bericht im Auftrag des Bundesrates,

International Trade Administration, U.S. Department of Commerce (2004): Pharmaceutical Price Controls in OECD Countries Implications for U.S. Consumers, Pricing, Research and Development, and Innovation, http://www.ita.doc.gov/td/health/DrugPricingStudy.pdf

Interpharma (2006): Pharmamarkt Schweiz, Ausgabe 2005, Basel

IMS Health (2006): Pricing and Market Access Review 2005, Cambridge, UK

IPSE: Parallel- und Reimporte von Arzneimitteln, Rechtliche Rahmenbedingungen in der Bundesrepublik Deutschland

Kanavos P. and Costa-Font J (2005): Pharmaceutical parallel trade in Europe: stakeholder and competition effects, Economic Policy October 2005, p 778

Knox, D, Richardson, M. (2002): Trade policy and parallel imports, European Journal of Political Economy Vol 19 (2002) 133–151, University of Otago, Dunedin, New Zealand

Läkemedelindustrieföreningen, LIF (2006): FAKTA 2006, Pharmaceutical Market and Health Care, Stockholm

Legemiddelindustrieforenigen, LMI (2002): Facts and Figures 2006: Medicines and Healthcare, Oslo, Norway, http://www.lmi.no/FullStory.aspx?m=146

Legemiddelindustrieforenigen, LMI (2006): Facts and Figures 2006: Medicines and Healthcare, Oslo, Norway, http://www.lmi.no/tf/2006/files/english/facts_and_figures_2006.pdf

Legemiddelindustrieforenigen, LMI (2007): Facts and Figures 2007: Medicines and Healthcare, Oslo, Norway, http://www.lmi.no/tf/2007/english/facts_and_figures_2007.pdf

Larsson. P (1999): Parallel Imports – Effects of the Silhouette Ruling, The Swedish Competition Authority, Stockholm

Maskus, K. E (2002): Vertical price control and parallel imports: theory and evidence, Washington D.C., The World Bank Group

Mepha Pharma AG (2005): Präsentation zur Jahres-Medienkonferenz, 03.02.2005

Mepha Pharma AG (2007): Präsentation zur Jahres-Medienkonferenz der Mepha-Gruppe, 19.01.2007

Morten Dalelen D. et al. (2006): Dag Morten Dalen et al. (2006), Price regulation and generic competition in the pharmaceutical market, University of Oslo, Health Economics Research Programme, Working Paper 2006.1

El Mundo (2005): Sanidad rebaja el precio de unos 4.500 medicamentos, 01.03.2005, http://www.elmundo.es/elmundosalud/2005/03/01/industria/1109675885.html, accessed 20.02.2006

Nguyen, N (1997): Physician behavioural response to a Medicare price reduction, Health Service Research

Pedersen K. et al. (2006): The economic impact of parallel import of pharmaceuticals, University of Southern Denmark, Odense

Poget, C. (2005): Are interventions in pharmaceutical markets an effective tool for cost containment? WWZ-Forschungsbericht, Basel

Reiffen D. and Ward M. (2002): Generic Drug Industry Dynamics, The Federal Trade Commission, Washingtom

Roth Johnsen J. (2006): Health Systems in Transition: Norway, Vol. 8 No. 1 2006, The European Observatory on Health Systems and Policies, Copenhagen, Denmark

Seydoux, Y (2005): Die schweizerische Bevölkerung bezahlt zu viel für Medikamente, Press Statement, Santésuisse, Solothurn

Swiss Federal Statistics Office (2005): Kosten und Finanzierung des Gesundheitswesens 2003, Neuchâtel

West P, Mahon. J (2002): Benefits to patients and payers from parallel trade, The York Health Economic Consortium

Vallgårda S. et al. (2001): Healthcare Systems in Transition: Denmark, Vol. 8, Nr. 7, The World Health Organization Regional Office for Europe, Copenhagen

Vaterlaus, S (2004): Auswirkungen eines Wechsels zur regionalen Erschöpfung im Patentrecht Aktualisierung und Ergänzung des Berichts «Erschöpfung von Eigentumsrechten: Auswirkungen eines Systemwechsels auf die schweizerische Volkswirtschaft», Plaut Economics, Berne

Vaterlaus, S (2002): Erschöpfung von Eigentumsrechten: Auswirkungen eines Systemwechsels auf die schweizerische Volkswirtschaft, Plaut Economics, Berne, Frontier Economics, London

Vaterlaus, S (2004): Warum erodieren Parallelimporte die Preisinsel Schweiz nicht stärker? Ermittlung der Rolle der geistigen Schutzrechte anhand exploratorischer Expertengespräche, Plaut Economics, Berne

VFA (2004): Reimporte: Kostendämpfung auf dem Irrweg, http://vfa.de/de/politik/artikelpo/reimporte.html, acceeded on 15.02.2006

Woodfield, A. (1999): Augmenting Reference Pricing of Pharmaceuticals with strategic cross-product agreements, University of Canterbury Working Paper, Christchurch, New Zealand

World Health Organization, (2002): Healthcare Systems in Transition: Switzerland, The World Health Organization, Copenhagen

World Trade Organisation: Agreement on Trade-Related Aspects of Intellectual Property Rights (TRIPS)

9.2   Interviews

Association of the British Pharmaceutical Industry (ABPI), Phil O'Neill, December 2nd, 2003

Eurim-Pharm, Andreas Mohringer, May 18th, 2004, Teleconference

European Federation of Pharmaceutical Industries Associations (EFPIA): François Bouvy, Brussels, November, 2003

Interpharma: Thomas Cueni, Heiner Sandmeier, Vincenza Trivigno, Basel, Multiple interviews 2002 through 2004

Lægemiddelindustriforeningen (Lif DK): Jørgen Clausen, Copenhagen, June 4th, 2004

Läkemedelsindustriföreningen, (LIF): Olle Hageberg, Teleconference, October, 2004

Legemiddelindustrieforenigen (LMI): Erik A. Stene, Per Olav Kormeset, Oslo, Novemeber 19th, 2004

Leo-Pharma: Jesper Noerregard, June 17th, 2004, Teleconference

Novartis (Pharma) AG: Martin Batzer, November 2003, Basel

Novartis International AG: Ernst Buser, October 2002, Basel

Orifarm (Danmark) A/S: Hans Bøgh-Sørensen, Thomas Brandhof, Ulrik Markussen, June 3rd, 2004

Orifarm (Sverige) AB: Fredrik Persson, Teleconference, May 26th, 2004

Pharos: Theo Berendsen, Barneveld (NL), June 21st 2004

Roche Deutschland Holding GmbH: Karl Schlingensief, Alexander Keusgen multiple interviews in 2003 and 2004

Roche Diagnostics (Deutschland) GmbH: Wulf-Fischer Knuppertz, Feruary 7th, 2004

Roche (Pharma) AG: Hans-Ruedi Wiedmer, René Imhof, Peter Heer, multiple interviews in 2003 and 2004

UCB Pharma: Christian Matton, Simon Loomann, Brussels, June 17th, 2004

Verband Forschender Arznemittelherstller (VFA): Walter Wittig, multiple interviews in 2003 and 2004

9.3   Statistical databases

Danish Medicine Agency (Lægemiddelstyrelsen): 5-year rolling pricing drug pricing database, all drugs grouped by ATC5 code, supplier, pack size, dosage, galenic form

Dansk Lægemiddel Information A/S: Sales and revenue information all ATC5 groups in Denmark, June 1999–July 2004, grouped by distribution channel (locally sourced or parallel traded)

EFPIA Statistics 2003: General Drug Market Statistics from all EFPIA member countries plus USA & Japan, data includes channel specific sales at pharmacy purchasing prices, R&D figures, basic pricing information

Farmastat AS: Sales Information: Sales and Revenue Information on 25 top selling products in Norway, pack specific data, grouped by product, dosage, pack size, galenic form and provider, annual (Oct 2004–Sep2003)

Läkemedelsstatistik AS: Sales and Revenue Information on 26 top selling products in Sweden, pack specific data, grouped by product, dosage, pack size, galenic form and provider, monthly January 2001–October 2004

OECD Health Data, 2003/2004/2005